RANDY HERRING

THE
FITNESS
MINDSET

7 HABITS FOR PEAK PERFORMANCE TO GET STRONG, LEAN, AND FIT

THE FITNESS MINDSET

*7 HABITS FOR PEAK PERFORMANCE
TO GET STRONG, LEAN, AND FIT*

To Shawnt -
Thank you for the great time
H₂O Water rafting ! Best
wishes in your endeavors!

By

Randy M. Herring

This book offers fitness and nutritional information and is designed for educational purposes only. Information contained herein is not a substitute for, nor does it replace, professional medical advice, diagnosis, or treatment. The use of any information provided on this book is solely at your own risk. Consult your physician or health care professional before starting any exercise program.

ISBN: 978-0-578-76119-0

For my boys Nasri and Shawn

with love…

CONTENTS

Contents (cont'd.)

THE FITNESS MINDSET

FOREWORD

Our Mindset creates the foundation of success in all areas of our lives. Whether a lens is low and wide to see a short distance or high and narrow to see a long distance, the lens in your own eye determines how you "see" yourself in relation toward success.

Mindset is built on values, habits and actions toward what is seen as possible. A mindset that excels for growth comes from a lens of abundance and opportunity. A mindset that surrenders to failure comes from a lens of scarcity and omission. Is your mind *set* on abundance and opportunity or scarcity and omission?

What we achieve in life is a measurement of what we value. Acquiring a fitness mindset to improve our functional performance and appearance is a difficult task, but like many things it is achieved by what we value and through repetitive acts.

Shifting from a "professional" frame of mind in our daily lives to a "fitness" frame of mind one hour a day is the same mind built from daily habits and behaviors than can help form and establish a fitness mindset. It takes small steps to build a fitness mindset, but one that inspires progress and opens the door to what is possible.

What sets those apart who master their training goals from those who don't are established values, habits and actions. Those who master their training goals wake up and "see" themselves actualizing their potential every day.

What every high performing person hears from others is, "I wish I had your commitment and strength" or "I couldn't do what you do." High performance habits are not easy to attain. We are not born with them. We must strive every day to hold on to them and strengthen them multiple times a day.

Both Randy and I share a strong commonality – a lifelong pursuit of fitness and over 20 years of experience as a certified personal trainer helping thousands of clients to tune into their mindset and reach their health and fitness goals.

Maybe you won't master your training goals fast. Maybe you won't shift your professional frame of mind to a fitness frame of mind easily. But where ever you are in your fitness journey, don't settle for less. Believe in what is possible. Aim high to perform well.

Read this book and learn how seven habits can help you train at a peak level and become unstoppable.

Jacques Pitcher
Team Pitcher Fitness Solutions
3x North American Masters Champion
National Physique Committee Judge

PREFACE

Mindset is influenced by external factors through life's experiences and learning from them. Mindset is nurtured – repeatedly.

Rewind 40 years.

When I was 15, I weighed a mere 115 pounds. I started lifting weights because I was bullied. I wanted to be stronger and have more confidence. I gained 55 pounds in eight months. In four months, I lost 25 pounds. In one year, I gained 30 pounds of muscle. I was more confident, stronger and bigger. I was ready to face my fears.

Fast forward 40 years. Older body. Stronger mind.

In January, a year before COVID-19, I looked into the mirror at the 56-year-old me and felt disgusted. My pants were tighter, I didn't feel good about myself and I wanted to feel and look better. I had to reclaim the bodybuilding-fitness lifestyle to transform my body and be healthy and in shape again.[1] I lost 17 pounds in the first 16 weeks and lost 25 pounds in a year. My confidence soared. I was stronger and leaner. I was ready to tell my story or at least that's what I thought.

Fast forward mid-March. COVID-19 2020 Pandemic.

I wasn't going to stop training and allow my body and mind turn to mush because of the mandated gym closures. I channeled my frustration and anger through the dark negative energy of the Pandemic by adapting to the circumstances and training hard with resistance tubes every morning. This gave me a single-pointed focus by responding to the stress of the Pandemic.

When the first lockdown was lifted after 51 days, I was stronger, more muscular and more defined. Bodybuilding gives me the resilience to fight back. It teaches me to persevere hardships and train hard to overcome them. I was ready to tell my story.

I am no Arnold Schwarzenegger. I am no Mat Fraser. I am no David Goggins. And I am certainly no titan. But like Arnold, bodybuilding put me on a path for better health and fitness.

I consider myself a normal guy in good athletic shape for my age. I am a cancer survivor – twice. My second round of cancer was a rare occurrence during my body transformation. But life-threatening setbacks can be overcome and can be minimal compared to the obstacles we face each day. Hard physical training can help you push through obstacles that life throws at you to make you stronger and more confident. I am telling you my story because I am confident that it can help you in some way.

The Fitness Mindset: 7 Habits For Peak Performance was first conceived out of my own personal body transformation within a year and a year before COVID-19. The book was conceived a second time, and when I actually began writing it, while I continued training during the course of the COVID-19 2020-21 Pandemic and Lockdowns from spring to winter.

This book was written for three reasons. One, how weight training can set you on a path for better health and fitness and manage your mind. Two, how exercising well can put you in tune with your body enabling you to perform at a peak level and give you the mindset to get the results you want. And three, how physical training can help you become resilient to overcome setbacks and push through obstacles every day whether they be physical, mental or psychological and make you strong again.

Building the body reaches out to the mind. The body obeys the mind because the mind controls what the body does. Therefore, mindset, the fourth habit, is related to habits affecting how we think and act, which controls the other six habits.

These other habits have to do with what and how often you eat, how well you are able to focus, how well you recover, how useful your exercise modality is, how well you are able to train for muscle tension and how well you are able to adapt your body to stress and transform itself. Each habit is a learnable skill you do repeatedly.

Look into the mirror of accountability, like I did, and take stock in your health and fitness. Now let's go. You've got this!

RMH

INTRODUCTION

A LIFELONG PURSUIT OF FITNESS

No question about it, sensible exercise is good for you. Yet, while we know it's in our best interests to exercise regularly, we find it too easy not to exercise.

Many people sacrifice their health for family, for friends, for a job, for wealth, or their happiness for these things, but do not put health as a priority to be rich. Good health gives you more time to enjoy life with the ones you love, travel more, build wealth and pursue the finer things in life. Healthy people often have long life expectancies, which give their investments time to grow. Good health is the least expensive investment you can give yourself.

Physical activity is a vital element of a healthy lifestyle. A sensible, balanced and consistent exercise program is good for the body. Movement is what we were meant to do. To meet the demands of life one needs to exercise their heart, lungs, muscles, bones, and joints to stay strong and healthy. We live, move and have our wellness through regular physical activity.

But the Information Age in which we live, along with its technological advances, has caused a decrease in physical activity. It has made us move less, eat more food, and expend less energy. The creation of online social platforms has exacerbated the problem. In the last 20 years healthcare costs have more than quadrupled due to a sedentary lifestyle with a lack of physical activity in the United States.[2]

According to the Center for Disease Control and Prevention (CDC), physical inactivity currently costs the United States $117 billion annually.[3] Statistics show that is costs much less to stay healthy and physically fit that it does to treat health ailments as a consequence of not living a healthy lifestyle.

The National Center for Biotechnology Information (NCBI) reports that diabetes and depression are highly prevalent in the United States. They are associated with increased mortality, lost work productivity, increased disability, decreased quality of life, and increased healthcare costs.[4]

Physical fitness improves the overall quality of life. It affects mood and mental state, physical appearance and performance, and brain activity. We engage in physical fitness for *psychological* reasons: to feel good about ourselves and have more confidence so that we can get things done and pursue other things in life that are worth enjoying (an activity, going out, taking a trip, etc.). We also engage in physical fitness for *physiological* and *neurological* reasons: to change physical appearance and increase functional ability (i.e., strength, muscle, endurance, coordination, flexibility) and to improve brain activity (i.e., cognition, focus, memory).

The benefits of physical fitness are incommensurable to any prescription, recreational drug, supplement or therapy can offer. Physical fitness contributes to positive thinking, increases confidence, metabolism, bone density, cardiovascular health, energy and hormones. It improves digestion, slows down the aging process, releases endorphins into the brain that reduce pain as a natural opiate and boost the feeling of well-being.

Studies show that exercise has the ability to reorganize and restructure brain activity called *neuroplasticity* as a treatment for depression.[5] Plasticity is creating new neurosynaptic connections by sending new and repeated signals to the brain, such as practicing a new physical activity. This repetitive action can "physically change" how one thinks because of the continued firing of learning new neurosynaptic pathways.[6] This means that increased physical activity improves mental performance and overall brain function.

Another study shows how the effect of exercise significantly reduces anxiety symptoms and chronic illness with prescribed training sessions lasting at least 30 minutes two times per week.[7] But this is not enough because this accounts for only 0.5% of the entire week.

When someone says he doesn't have time to exercise what he is really saying is that he doesn't place a high value on his health to be motivated to exercise. But this may not be entirely his fault. Like a lot of people, he probably doesn't have a plan to help him decide on a goal so that he can take action to be healthier and have the know-how to strive toward a goal.

And if someone wants to lose weight but is following a strength training plan, then losing weight is to no avail. It is because the goal doesn't match the training plan. And the same thing with gaining muscle. If someone wants to gain muscle but is following a strength training plan, then gaining muscle is without success since the goal doesn't match the training plan. Once you've committed yourself to a goal a fitness plan must meet that goal to achieve it.

A physical fitness plan must include the following three exercise components: (1) training, (2) nutrition and (3) recuperation. Training can create the proper environment during exercise to *stimulate* change (to your body). Nutrition can aid recovery after exercise to *promote* change. And recuperation can help the body become stronger and increase performance after exercise to *effect* change.

According to the National Health and Nutrition Examination Survey (NHANES), as reported by the CDC, 74% American adults over 20 years old are overweight and obese.[8] The CDC also reported that 23% of American adults participate in physical exercise 60 minutes four times per week.[9, 10] It seems logical to conclude that the remaining 3% account for American adults engaged in physical fitness 60 to 90 minutes five to seven days a week.

But this doesn't mean that 3% are engaged in improving their fitness. It means that 3% have built physical fitness into a daily habitual routine, however, presupposing that 2% do not improve their fitness because they can be seen by "going through the motions," whereas an elite 1% are visually immersed in their work because they train with a purpose through hard physical training.

Thus, it is reasonable to say that 99% people fail without trying to improve their health and fitness or do not reach their fitness goals because they don't have a training plan or one that is enjoyable, have unrealistic expectations, and lack accountability. Instead, it seems as if this 99% want to be given the magic formula, the answer that will make them healthier, stronger, and fitter. There are three problems with this.

First of all, there are many ways a person can become healthy and fit. With the birth of the Internet, experts have been created to stir you towards the best way to build a better body. But each person needs to find what exercise modality works best for him or her and one that is enjoyable.

The second problem is that people who look for a magic formula can fall prey to marketing tactics that sell magic formulas, such as, "Lose weight fast, guaranteed!" The third problem is that most people cannot follow a formula for long, which is why, for example, there are so many different diet and fitness programs being sold, generally to the same people.

The Fitness Mindset reveals why 99% do not reach their fitness goals. It is because they are focused on the end goal, the result, rather than the continual process of exercising and repeating a fitness plan that progressively builds up a good habit that can stimulate, promote and effect changes and transform the whole body.

Physical fitness is a personal journey. It requires your heart. It takes time. It involves patience. It claims self-respect. It is hard because it commands a plan and demands perseverance.

To promote one's health and fitness the mind must be engaged in the activity of an exercise. The Greek philosopher, Aristotle, tells us that activities are made more enjoyable by their corresponding proper pleasures.[11] The proper pleasure to promote health is perspiration. That is, if one wishes to exercise as the cause to promote health, then one will perspire as a particular effect.

Aristotelian and Catholic theologian, St. Thomas Aquinas, sheds light on this. He says that since exercising is a worthy activity and, therefore, good to promote health – "knowing beforehand [we] will work up a sweat" – it follows that we will perspire as the cause to promote health as a particular effect.[12] Thus, the proper pleasure to the activity of an exercise is sweating. In other words, sweating is the cause of *exercising* to promote health to a greater degree.

Furthermore, when we enjoy exercising very much, "we do not throw ourselves into anything else, and do [this] one thing only."[13] As a result, we will sweat more because our body has become more efficient by *learning how* to exercise well and, thus, makes the exercise more precise to meet the end goal.

However, when a person finds exercise to unpleasant, he will seek what Aristotle describes as "alien pleasures."[14] Alien pleasures are contrary to the activity because they destroy the proper pleasure to exercising, i.e., sweating. Since this person is disconnected by the activity that he finds to be unpleasant, he invites contrary pleasures to enter his mind, such as reading a book, looking through social media, listening to a pod cast, watching TV, looking around the gym, etc. The consequence of this is that he may or may not promote his health and fitness, and if he does, to a lesser degree.

Transformations of every sort cannot occur without learning to build a strong mind and having a *raison d'être* (reason to be) in your heart. Proverbs says, "As a man thinks in his heart, so he is" (23:7). Learning to build a strong mind is a repetitive skill. To be the change you want to see requires you to do something about it repeatedly to be the cause of it. A strong mind is the cause of a transformation and a stronger mind causes subsequent transformations.

You are what you do repeatedly. Developing good healthy habits takes time to ground as "second nature." Believe in yourself, train intelligently, be patient and you will see results. Each day, each month, and each year is a new starting point. Focus on the process of change and not the end goal itself. When you focus on the process toward the goal, the prize will come.

The chapters in this book are organized by key words from each subsequent letter of the word F-O-R-M-U-L-A (with exception of the last chapter) that describes each of the seven habits. Each chapter begins with a short sentence in italics describing the habit or what each habit stands for.

For example, the first habit in Chapter 1 is "food," and "f" is the first letter in the word formula. The second habit in Chapter 2 is "optimal," and "o" is the second letter in the word formula. The third habit in Chapter 3 is "recover," and "r" is the third letter in the word formula and so on with "mindset," "useful," "limitless" and "adaptation." Chapters 1, 3, 5-8 deal with the physiology of exercise and functioning at a higher level. And chapters 2 and 4 deal with the psychology of exercising and performing at an optimal level.

Each chapter is divided into sections. Some chapters have many sections while others have only a few. The table of contents list only three sections under each chapter what it highlights.

Chapter 1 addresses the importance of nutrition in conjunction with exercise, and emphasizes the latter since exercise influences healthier food choices. This chapter also provides a few words on water, alcohol and caffeine, and suggests various macronutrient ratios to aid in reaching a particular goal. Chapter 2 extracts the importance of the Self and introduces the concept 'flow,' which is described as a skill called "flow experiences" to enhance exercise focus for peak performing workouts. This chapter, you might say, was written in part in the gym. Chapter 3 discusses recuperation after exercise and what the exercise enthusiast must do to help increase functional performance.

Chapter 4 talks about three mindsets but only one that knows how to train with the right routine, the right amount of intensity, the right form, and eat the right amounts of foods at the right time and often enough in order to perform at a peak level to attain a goal. Valuation excuses are introduced that we tend to talk ourselves into believing that only limit possibilities. I recount how Arnold Schwarzenegger can put you on a quest to adapt to every environment and train first-rate anywhere and anyhow. Believe that power is fueled from within, transformations are innate and miracles do happen!

Chapter 5 compares weight training to various high-impact exercise modalities. Other topics include the importance of muscle tension, training techniques you can do by yourself to make workouts more productive, injuries and injury prevention, body types and training plans, full-body vs split routines, and what it means to exercise well.

Chapter 6 distinguishes between three weight training methods. The third qualifies as the best and most useful approach. Overtraining is briefly discussed after the first method because of the tendency to train too much. Other topics include high-volume vs high-intensity training systems, measuring "time under tension," and the importance of warming-up.

Chapter 7 discusses how the same workout routine can get you results. The desire to "change up" your routine citing that a "plateau" has been reached is based on the assumption that every nutrition and training variable has been exhausted. The exerciser is challenged to re-evaluate his or her training on two criteria as to why results have come to a standstill.

Chapter 8 teaches you how to exercise more effectively by understanding the planes of motion, joint movement, muscle function and joint alignment. Knowing how the limbs on the body move and how the muscles function in relation to that movement and joint alignment with other joints can make an exercise safe and effective and help you train intelligently to get results.

This book concludes with three Appendices. Appendices A and B are my full-body resistance and cardio routines pre-COVID-19 2020 lockdown and COVID-19 2020 lockdown. Appendix C lists a few of my favorite high protein and low carb recipe dishes.

CHAPTER 1

OPTIMIZE YOUR FOOD RATIO

Optimize your food ratio to promote change in functional performance and body composition.

You are what you eat (or don't eat). There are tens of thousands of diets registered with the *American Dietetic Association*, yet half the population of the United States remain overweight. This is because on a calorie deprivation diet most of the weight lost is muscle, which results in a slower metabolism and more fat. Having a higher ratio of muscle to fat to total body mass weight is fundamental for a higher metabolism to lose fat. Muscle is essentially your fat burning machinery.

The 'Diet' Craze

Do diets work? On the outset we are inclined to say, no. But it all depends on how 'diet' is defined, what kind of diet it is, and why (for what purpose) it is used. The conventional usage of diet means to deprive the body of essential nutrients needed for maintenance and repair (protein) and fuel (carbohydrates).

Any diet that proposes rapid weight reduction (including muscle and water) are "crash" diets and nothing but fads, farces and lies. In the end, the creators of these diets become wealthy and the dieter, who are usually sedentary individuals, becomes less healthy than before.

If diet is rightly defined as a "newly acquired eating behavior" (and not one that is temporary), then the goal of any sensible diet should be to educate one to *assume healthier eating habits that is sustainable to effectively manage weight.* When you adopt a lifestyle of overall health and fitness then your weight balances naturally. My diet plan consists of five to six daily meals. I spend at least 2 to 4 hours a week making dishes for the week so my meals are already prepped and ready to eat.

Diet and Exercise

The body's metabolism decreases by 3% each year known as "creeping obesity." I discovered that my metabolism slows down every five years, which started at the age of 41. It slowed down at 46 and also 51. My body transformation began shortly after realizing the most recent metabolic decrease at 56.

The good news is that metabolic decreases can be offset by a change in lifestyle with an exercise *and* diet plan. When an effective weight resistance exercise routine is used in conjunction with diet, the body's metabolism remains elevated four to seven days after exercise.

Cardiorespiratory exercise, in comparison, only elevates the body's metabolism 24 to 48 hours after exercise. Furthermore, studies have shown that exercise alone, compared to dieting alone, is more effective for weight management.

A Holistic Ratio

The 80/20 rule is a myth. Getting results by altering physical appearance and improving functional ability is not 80% nutrition and 20% exercise, but quite the opposite: 80% exercise and 20% nutrition.

Consider this: You spend 2 to 4 hours a week "meal prepping," whereas you spend 7 to 10 hours a week "exercising." Meal prepping makes up 2% of our entire week, whereas exercising makes up 4 to 6% of our entire week. After you prep your meals all you have to do is eat. Exercising takes more time (and effort), even in preparation.

But the reason why most people have heard that getting results is 80% nutrition and 20% exercise is that this ratio is used in reference to a bodybuilder's lifestyle: eat, train, sleep, repeat.

Training is relatively the easy part for a bodybuilder because it is a pleasurable activity compared to around the clock high-performance nutrition to help with recovery and increase performance in the gym and change body composition.

The latter ratio must be applied to the majority who do not find exercise pleasurable and do not adhere to the regimen of a bodybuilder. An 80% exercise and 20% nutrition ratio must realistically apply to a domestic 9-5 lifestyle: work, home, sleep, repeat.

Living a domestic lifestyle makes it more difficult to make exercise a priority in order to make it a habit and exercise well. Learning how to exercise well by allowing the body to adapt and, therefore, change is not 20%, but 80% (given the perspective that movement is what we were meant to do throughout our lifetime).

Learning how to exercise well takes time, which is how habits are formed. When a training session is more difficult to get through it is likely the case that one did not eat high-performance nutrition in regard to the right foods in the right amounts at the right time and often enough to allow the body to recover for the next training session.

This recovery period, although ongoing throughout the day and night, would in fact constitute 80%. Eating high-performance nutrition meals definitely increases exercise performance and invariably aids in a series of body transformations. The bottom line is that when one exercises (first), then one will make healthier food choices (second) in order to perform and function better (third). Studies show that exercising influences healthier eating.[15] Movement (exercise) comes first, and eating better (diet) comes second.

However, when we talk about an 80/20 ratio that is 80% exercise and 20% nutrition, we should be pragmatic and talk about a holistic 34/33/33 ratio that includes all three components (training, nutrition, recovery) working together to increase performance and improve the body. We should, therefore, speak of a 34% exercise, 33% nutrition, and 33% recovery ratio.

Eat 4-6 Small Frequent Meals

Food breaks down as energy to fuel and repair the body and assist in its functioning. It is fundamental to fuel the body with a nutritious food or drink an hour to an hour and a half before exercise in order to provide the necessary energy to fuel a workout. This creates the proper training environment to stimulate changes to the body.

When a person limits food intake the body's metabolism decreases. A slower metabolism has the propensity to increase fat mass. The solution to increase the body's metabolism is to eat 4-6 frequent meals a day.

Eating small frequent meals is important because it: (1) helps the body to utilize nutrients more effectively and efficiently, (2) promotes satiety to avoid over-eating, and (3) helps boost metabolism and maintain energy levels. If you have been eating 1-2 meals a day for many years, then it is realistic to add another meal a day while slowly working up to 4-6 meals daily in conjunction with regular exercise.

Food has the effect of increasing the body's metabolism because the body releases energy to digest and absorb the nutrients. In addition, eating small frequent meals daily aids in the recovery process after exercise to promote change from minutes to hours to days. We eat for energy. So, let's use it.

Drink Water Between Meals

Water is the oxygen of life. Human beings can go without food for nearly a month, but without water for only a few days.

Bottled water is the most consumed beverage on the planet next to caffeinated drinks. The bottled water industry is a profitable and lucrative business generating nearly 20 billion dollars in annual sales. But nearly 3 billion people experience water shortage, which is why our water supply is in trouble.[16, 17]

The body is made up of 60% water. Muscles are primarily composed of about 72% water by weight. So, if you are looking for a swollen pump during your workout, drink lots of water! Water also aids in fat metabolism. If you want to lose weight, then drink plenty of water.

Drinking anywhere from 8 to 16 glasses of water daily is the recommendation. Drinking lots of water means you'll be making frequent trips to the bathroom at night until your body adjusts.

When your pee is clear it means that your urinary system and kidneys are flushing out toxic wastes and poisons from the body. The least inexpensive "body cleanse" I can think of is a water cleanse.

Drinking a lot of water with meals may interfere with the digestion and absorption of nutrients because it can dilute them. So, it is best to drink water primarily between meals. The absorption of nutrients is necessary for repair of the muscles and recovery for the whole body after a workout. In addition, thirst is a poor indication that you need water. Thirst actually indicates that you've been dehydrated for quite some time.

The Contested Enhancement of Caffeine[18]

Caffeine is available to everyone and socially acceptable. It is generally safe in moderate amounts (65 to 400mg) with an average daily consumption of 200mg. Caffeine is classified as a psychoactive stimulant mood-altering drug. It is the most widely consumed drug found predominately in coffee.

Coffee is the leading beverage consumed worldwide after water. The coffee industry revenues are at least three times more than bottled water because of the average cost difference. Starbucks is by far the largest coffee house chain worldwide. The average cost of a 16.9 oz bottled water currently costs $0.70 whereas a Starbucks freshly brewed medium coffee costs $2.10.[19]

Caffeine is not only found in coffee and latte's (100-320mg per 8-16 oz cup) but also in sport "energy" drinks (48-300mg per 8-16 oz can), soft drinks (30-72mg per 12 oz serving), "weight loss" supplements (100-300mg per tablet or capsule), chewing gum (30-100mg per stick), pills (100-200mg per tablet), water (34-125mg per 12-16.9 oz can or bottle) and powder.[20]

Caffeine primarily affects the central nervous system (CNS) and the brain. Caffeine triggers the release of adrenalin for increased energy and may increase fat metabolism, enhance cognitive skills and improve work and exercise performance. Triggering the release of adrenalin is brief and temporary. Everything that speeds up must invariably slow down. The increased energy (and rise in high blood pressure and heart rate) is real, but "feeling" the effects of caffeine to lose weight, enhance skills or perform better might possibly be a placebo effect.

Consuming a moderate amount of caffeine may lead to health risks because of the potential of taking excessive amounts due to prolonged use. Health risks include: rapid heart rate (tachycardia), high blood pressure (hypertension), mood alteration, anxiety disorder, restlessness, insomnia, stomach and intestinal pain, fatigue and probable addiction.

Discontinuing caffeine results in a "crash." Withdrawal symptoms include: headache, muscle aches and pains, lethargy, irritability, loss of concentration and in severe cases can lead to depression and suicidal thinking. To prevent the crash from occurring the recommendation is to ingest caffeine at appropriate times to preserve the body's caffeinated physiological equilibrium.

Arguments for caffeine is that it is derived from nature. Therefore, it is permissible to use it to improve our nature and performance. Arguments against caffeine is that it interferes with the body's natural function ability. This raises questions about the moral status of nature and the ethics of human enhancement. Therefore, it is not permissible to use caffeine since it alters the psych and affects a decline of the body and health.

Seeking to enhance our natural dispositions by ingesting caffeine might seem un-existential, and in the opinion of Briggle, "is a bad case of bad faith – unsure of who we are, but certain that we are supposed to be happy."[21]

But let's get real. Most of us cannot live without caffeine. People drink coffee for the taste and smell along with its mild to extreme stimulating benefits either for social occasions or our daily energy. People who do not drink coffee take a pill for the moderate to extreme stimulating effects.

Make a value judgment. People drink or take caffeine to enhance their lives by functioning and performing better, which causes them to "live better." But what goes up must come down. Does caffeine provide sustainable energy and a stable mood that might hold for a "better" life? Now make a psychological valuation.

If caffeine has such a downswing, then what keeps us on the upswing? Caffeine? No, it can't and doesn't. Exercise keeps us on the upswing. Physical activity (walking), physical exercise (cycling), and physical fitness (weight training, TRX, functional training, spartan races, titan games, etc.) is energy sustaining and psychologically motivating.

An exercise routine along with a sensible meal plan provides a natural long-lasting effect that caffeine doesn't offer: sustained energy, increased cognitive skills, improved functional ability and enhanced performance. A healthy and more fit lifestyle can give a greater sense of well-being and feeds our wellness by empowering us daily. It is not how one lives better, but how one lives well.

Alcoholic Beverages

Alcohol is a depressant and legal drug. It is absorbed into the body in several places. About 20 to 40 percent of the alcohol is absorbed into the stomach. The remaining 60 to 80 percent of the alcohol leaves the stomach and moves into the small intestine and into the bloodstream. This is when the effects of alcohol become noticeable. Because alcohol is water-based, it is absorbed very quickly.

Alcohol affects the central nervous system (CNS) and the brain. Alcohol causes deterioration of body functions, of judgement, of self-control and disrupts transmission of sensory impulses from the brain to the muscles.

There are no benefits to drinking alcohol. One, alcohol is poison to the body. Two, alcohol destroys nutrients. Three, alcohol causes dehydration. Four, alcohol slows down recuperation. Five, alcohol inhibits fat metabolism. And six, alcohol contributes to laying down and storing more fat.

Optimize Your Nutrient Food Ratios

Optimizing carbohydrates, protein and fat amounts per meal and per day using macronutrient ratios are nothing new. Bodybuilders have been perfecting their diets to build or get lean by adjusting their protein, carbohydrates and fat intake for years before they were known as "macronutrient ratios" (MNRs). So, when people utilize MNRs, they are in a sense adopting a part of a body-*building* or body-*sculpting* nutrition regimen to attain a goal.[22]

Do not count calories. Count macronutrients (carbohydrates, protein, fat) since they make up total calories. The primary function of *carbohydrates* is to provide energy. The primary function of *protein* is to build, maintain, and repair tissues. And the primary function of *fat* is to assist in body functions and promote satiety.

Carbohydrates yield 4 calories per gram. It is the primary source of fuel for the body at 1,600 calories per pound. Protein yields 4 calories per gram. It is a secondary source of fuel for the body at 2,000 calories per pound. And fat yields 9 calories per gram. It is the third and last source of fuel for the body at 3,500 calories per pound.

I learned about MNRs as a personal trainer at the turn of the millennium. At the time it included five profile types that most people fell under in regard to what foods they normally ate and what MNR was recommended. Since then, these five profile types have been discarded. Profile 3 was considered the average profile what macronutrient foods people frequently ate.

Optimizing your MNRs do not tell you *what* to eat, only a range *where* you should be at +/-5% of each macronutrient.[23] The ratio percentages have since been modified as seen in the profile chart below compared to the generalized chart on the next page.

Profile	Protein	Carbohydrate	Fat
1	15%	75%	10%
2	20%	65%	15%
3	20%	60%	20%
4	20%	55%	25%
5	25%	45%	30%

Preliminary Orientation to Food Ratios

Consuming 175 grams of protein yields 700 protein calories (175 x 4). Consuming 350 grams of carbohydrates yields 1400 carbohydrate calories (350 x 4). Consuming 80 grams of fat yields 720 fat calories (80 x 9). Total calories: 2,820. Now the percentages. Protein: 700 / 2820

= 25%. Carbohydrates: 1400 / 2820 = 50%. Fat: 720 / 2820 = 25%. The percentages would constitute the following macronutrient ratio: 25% protein / 50% carbohydrates / 25% fat. This is a very good and sustainable ratio for most people when combined with exercise.

Macronutrient	Recommendation range percent of total calories
Carbohydrates	50-70%
Protein	15-30%
Fat	10-30%

The basic rule is that to build muscle you must move less for a surplus of calories. To lose fat you must move more for a deficit of calories. To build muscle *and* lose fat you must find a balance between moving more and moving less, but leaning toward moving more, since the primary objective is to "lean out." To build strength and muscle *and* lose fat you must incorporate a lot of compound movements and eat more to have a surplus of calories to build muscle, which is necessary for fat loss.

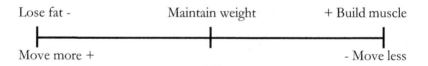

A safe and effective fat loss should be no more than 4 pounds per month. More would constitute muscle loss. An effective muscle gain should be no more than 2 pounds per month. Fat losses and muscle gains will always be greater at the start of an exercise program and slow down thereafter but you can still make improvements. A Chinese proverb says, "Do not be afraid of moving slowly; only be afraid of standing still."

The suggested nutrient ratios below relate to a specific body composition goal but do not take into consideration gender, age, activity level, basal metabolic rate (BMR) or the body's energy expenditure at rest and body composition. Follow a food ratio or create one that best suits your body and desired goal.

Sedentary Person: Maintain Muscle and Fat

A suggested ratio to *maintain muscle and fat* a sedentary individual weighing 180 pounds would consume at least 0.6 grams of protein, 1.5 grams of carbohydrates, and 0.2 grams of fat per pound of body weight. This would consist of 108 grams of protein (432 calories), 270 grams of carbohydrates (1,080 calories), and 36 grams of fat (324 calories) totaling 1,836 calories. The ratio would look like this: 23% protein / 59% carbohydrates / 18% fat.

Physically Active Person: Decrease Fat and Maintain Muscle

A suggested ratio to *decrease fat and maintain muscle* a physically active person weighing 200 pounds with 14% body fat would consume 0.9 grams of protein per pound of muscle weight, 1.8 grams of carbohydrates per pound of body weight, and 0.3 grams of fat per pound of body weight. This would consist of 155 grams of protein (620 calories), 360 grams of carbohydrates (1,440 calories), and 60 grams of fat (540 calories) for a total of 2,600 calories (assuming this caloric intake is 300-500 below maintenance calories). The ratio would look like this: 24% protein / 55% carbohydrate / 21% fat. This is an excellent ratio.

Recreational Bodybuilder: Build Muscle and Decrease Fat

A suggested ratio to *build muscle and decrease fat* a recreational bodybuilder (a person who engages in bodybuilding fitness training, but doesn't compete) weighing 200 pounds with 14% body fat would consume 1.5 grams of protein per pound of muscle weight, 0.3 grams of carbohydrates per pound of body weight, and 0.5 grams of fat per pound of body weight. This would consist of 258 grams of protein (1032 calories), 60 grams of carbohydrates (240 calories), and 100 grams of fat (900 calories) for a total of 2,172 calories. The ratio would look like this: 48% protein / 11% carbohydrate / 41% fat.

Recreational Bodybuilder: Build Muscle and Maintain Fat (1)

A suggested ratio to *build muscle and maintain fat* a recreational bodybuilder weighing 180 pounds with 6% body fat would consume 1 gram of protein per pound of muscle weight, 2.5 grams of carbohydrates per pound of body weight, and 0.4 grams of fat per pound of body weight. This would consist of 169 grams of protein (676 calories), 450 grams of carbohydrates (1,800 calories), and 72 grams of fat (648 calories) for a total of 3,124 calories. The ratio would look like this: 22% protein / 57% carbohydrates / 21% fat.

A fat ratio between 20-25% is good for building muscle. But a decrease in fat below 10% and/or an increase of protein above 30% of total calories is not recommended unless you are training for a bodybuilding competition. In addition, a high-protein consumption can tax the kidneys, which go into overdrive trying to process and excrete the nitrogen in protein. To compensate for this drink plenty of water. Drinking up to a gallon or 4 liters or more of water per day between meals helps with the transportation of important nutrients for muscular growth.

Recreational Bodybuilder: Build Muscle and Maintain Fat (2)

A suggested ratio to *build muscle and maintain fat* a recreational bodybuilder weighing 200 pounds with 14% body fat would consume 1 gram of protein per pound of muscle weight, 2.5 grams of carbohydrates per pound of body weight, and 0.4 grams of fat per pound of body weight. This would consist of 172 grams of protein (688 calories), 500 grams of carbohydrates (2,000 calories), and 80 grams of fat (720 calories) for a total of 3,408 calories (assuming this caloric intake is 300-500 above maintenance calories). The ratio would look like this: 20% protein / 59% carbohydrate / 21% fat.

When I trained consistently while living in Japan, I decreased my fat intake as low as 5% of my total calories. But I didn't compensate my body for this by increasing my protein and carbohydrate intake to replace my lowered fat intake. The result was that I lost a great deal of muscle.

Endurance Athlete: Maintain Muscle

A suggested ratio to *maintain muscle* an endurance athlete weighing 180 pounds with 10% body fat would consume 1 gram of protein per pound of muscle weight, 3.5 grams of carbohydrates per pound of body weight, and 0.3 grams of fat per pound of body weight. This would consist of 162 grams of protein (648 calories), 630 grams of carbohydrates (2,520 calories), and 54 grams of fat (486 calories) for a total of 3,654 calories. The ratio would look like this: 18% protein / 69% carbohydrates / 13% fat.

HABIT #1

Optimize Your Food Ratio to Promote Change

Summary Chart

Level of Activity	Desired Goal	Macronutrient Recommendations
Sedentary	Maintain muscle and fat	0.6 gms protein per lb muscle, 1.5 gms carbs & 0.2 gms fat per lb body wt.
Physically Active	Decrease fat / Maintain muscle	0.9 gms protein per lb muscle, 1.8 gms carbs & 0.3 gms fat per body wt.

For a physically active female over 35% body fat adjust the carbohydrate intake to 0.9; for a physically active male over 22% body fat adjust it to 1.5

Recreational bodybuilder	Build muscle / Decrease fat	1.5 gm protein per lb muscle, 0.3 gms carbs & 0.5 gms fat per lb body wt.
Recreational bodybuilder (1) & (2)	Build muscle / Maintain fat	1 gm protein per lb muscle, 2.5 gms carbs & 0.4 gms fat per lb body wt.
Recreational bodybuilder	Maintain muscle / Decrease fat	1.3 gm protein per lb muscle, 0.5 gms carbs & 0.7 gms fat per lb body wt.
Competitive bodybuilder	Build muscle / Maintain fat	2 gms protein, 2.5 gms carbs & 0.2 gms fat per lb body wt.
Competitive bodybuilder	Decrease fat / Maintain muscle	1.5 gms protein, 1.8 gms carbs & 0.2 gms fat per lb body wt.

Competitive bodybuilding may require extremely more protein and less carbohydrates especially if the desired goal is to increase muscle and decrease fat.

Endurance athlete	Maintain muscle	1 gm protein per lb muscle, 3.5 gms carbs & 0.3 gms fat per lb body wt.

CHAPTER 2

THE FLOW OF EXERCISING

The flow of exercising enables you to train at an optimal *level unimpeded by contrary pleasures so you can focus to accomplish a specific task.*

German philosopher Friedrich Nietzsche is representative of what could be called a "philosophy of life." Life, for him, is a process of self-discovery and the power to "become what one is."[24] Nietzsche insisted that life is not meaningless. Life is good and embracing hardships is essential for "becoming" who you are.

Be Yourself!

The journey of self-discovery is one of the greatest difficulties, yet the greatest reward in life to achieve happiness. Nietzsche says, "Every human being is a unique miracle...beautiful, and worth regarding."[25] He echoes Emerson's words verbatim, "'all experiences are useful, all days holy and all people divine'!!!"[26]

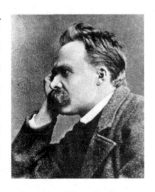

Nietzsche's philosophy of life is rigorous like tough physical training possessing a kind of athletic mindset. To discover and actualize the essence of your "existential" being you must overcome that which negates the actual self. Negative thoughts negate becoming. Positive thoughts affirm becoming. We choose our frame of mind. Discovering your true authentic self is tough. It is a process of deconstructing your life to understand the relationship between you and the world and life's meaning. It is a challenging and frightening process because social media has us sucked into its vacuum day in and day out to pacify our need to belong to an esteemed group and make us feel loved through an emoji affirmation. The unconscious self struggles to affirm the authentic self because it is caught in between the social web of the "adverse" self – what it is not. "All that you are now doing, thinking, desiring," Nietzsche says, "is not you, yourself."[27] Discovering your true authentic self is an everyday constant self-overcoming of your adverse self.

Discovering your authentic self is to suffer *through* it with hard physical and mental labor. But it doesn't stop there. After you "discover" yourself, you must seek to overcome a part of yourself that tries to dissuade you from striving toward the goal of becoming a better and stronger you. It is a difficult task, but is the greatest reward, the prize of life. This is happiness. It is freedom.

Nietzsche's formula of happiness resides in his concept of the Overman or Superman.[28] The sheer magnificence of the existence of life is embracing its joys and hardships. We should be happy and learn to love the choices we make (good and bad) and be our own heroes by affirming them wholeheartedly. To turn "muck into gold" is to master hardships and overcome them and become self-overcomers.[29]

Nietzschean happiness is not relying on externally driven goals that society sets before us as means to an end, but internally driven goals that you value for their own sake to make life more rich, intense and meaningful. It is a path that you set and create yourself. There is no universal path. It is a path that can be dark and frightening because there are no blueprints. It is a rigorous and narrow yet fluid path. It is your path and your life. This is happiness.[30] Suffering through hardships is the key to unlocking the secret of happiness. Happiness is not in opposition to pain and exertion. It is rather striving toward something in suffering through a great task you've set yourself. Overcoming obstacles is part of the experience of happiness. It is not just pleasure, but pain that can be happiness. Pain is almost an enabling condition of happiness.[31]

Nietzsche admonishes, "Any human being who does not wish to belong to the masses needs only to stop taking things easy for himself. Let him follow his conscience, which calls to him: *Be yourself!*"[32]

Repetition and Commitment

Aristotle says, "It is from the repeated performance of right actions that we become good."[33] One action or one brief space of time does not make a person true and good, but repeated acts.[34] And likewise with discovering yourself. One act of self-discovery does not mean you've discovered who you are, but repeated self-overcoming acts to assert your true authentic self.

Will Durant paraphrases Aristotle, "Excellence is an art won by training and habituation. We do not act rightly because we have virtue or excellence, but we rather have those because we have acted rightly. We are what we repeatedly do. Excellence, then, is not an act but a habit."[35]

If your task is to become a good human being, then you will do good acts all the time. If your task is to become who you are, then you will labor to overcome yourself every day. If your task is to become healthy, then you will be active always. If your task is to become physically fit, then you will train and eat right daily.

"You are what you repeatedly do" means you are engaged and committed to a great task staying on the path that leads to the goal that you have set for yourself – to be yourself.

The Objective Necessity of Selfishness[36]

Often selfishness is considered to be a negative concept, especially when it is referenced in relation to something else. For example, selfishness is "concern with one's own interest *in* disregard of others." This definition *does* render it negative because of the subjective reference it creates with the preposition *in*. This is how it can be considered negative.

But when you approach the word on its own term without any reference in relation to something else it is purely defined objectively and renders it good: "concern with one's own interest." Let me explain.

Selfishness established as *concern with one's own interest* translates into *self-love*. It is having behavior towards yourself that is loving. We think of positive words like growth, opportunity, create, produce, even love itself. A prerequisite to becoming not just anyone but someone is selfishness. Good things cannot be achieved that can benefit yourself and others without first becoming selfish and having a purpose – a *rational selfishness.*

A rational self-interest is taking care of yourself. It is taking care of your health. This is not only good for you, but also good for all. For choosing better health, as a value to love yourself, it becomes a value for all who are concerned. Better health is not only good for you, but also good for everyone to whom can *gain advantage* of countless health-related *benefits.*

This is what I mean by the objective necessity of selfishness in reference to health and fitness. So, if you want to get healthy and fit or get better at doing something and excel in it you first must be selfish in your pursuit.

There is nothing better than to have a strong, healthy and fit body that you have worked your ass off you can call your own and love. This self-serving achievement displays feelings of self-satisfaction because it is self-respecting and self-demanding. In the last analysis selfishness is pronounced good, blessed and holy.

Goals, Values and Motivation

Achieving a goal leads to self-satisfaction and self-worth. Failing to achieve a goal, can lead to self-censure. Now, to achieve a goal that is highly valued one must have a hierarchical order of goals from less valued goals to highly valued goals. Less valued goals are subgoals, whereas highly valued goals are superordinate goals. Achieving subgoals gets you closer to achieving superordinate goals.[37] For example, if your superordinate goal is to be fit, then you must join a gym, workout and exercise more.

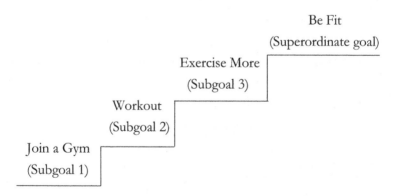

Be Fit
(Superordinate goal)

Exercise More
(Subgoal 3)

Workout
(Subgoal 2)

Join a Gym
(Subgoal 1)

Superordinate goals are higher-ordered and long-term goals that are more intrinsically valued because they are tied to our self-worth. Subgoals are lower-ordered and short-term goals that are less valued and can be given up more easily. But subgoals provide benchmarks by which to measure your progress towards the more distant superordinate goals.[38] Meeting subgoals daily is a process for getting you closer to achieving superordinate goals.

Our action to reach a superordinate goal depends on our self-evaluative reactions to our behavior for the successes (self-worth) and failures (self-censure) and the strength of value placed on the goal to motivate us to achieve it.[39] The value placed on a goal assumes a person believes that the desired outcome can be achieved by acting. If the person believes he is not capable of achieving the outcome, he will have little motivation to act and self-regulate.[40] The belief in one's capabilities to execute action required to manage a situation *and* succeed is called "self-efficacy," which can either strengthen or undermine one's motivation to engage in self-regulation.[41] This is why believing in yourself matters.

Motivation comes from within. It is fueled by the desire to maintain a value to achieve a goal. A goal that is achieved is more valued and will be given more motivation to strive to meet another goal and so on. That motivation is in the *activity itself* and manifests the value of that striving because of feelings of self-satisfaction.[42] And the motivation of striving to meet a goal that is more valued requires the skills to achieve it.[43] 'Flow' is a concept that can make the present activity more enjoyable because it builds the self-confidence that allows to develop the skills of training to make exercising fun, effective and rewarding.

Flow Experiences[44]

Having peak performing workouts comes from the exercise of skills you repeatedly do. The motivation of the activity itself to train at a peak level is the self-satisfaction of the skill that produces it. The skill that produces peak level training is called "flow experiences."[45] These experiences help you exercise well so you can transition over to performing at an optimal level.

Doing repeated instances of flow experiences enable you to focus single-pointedly on the *immediate task* of training on a particular exercise movement at that moment and have an optimal exercise experience. Flow experiences will help you produce peak performing workouts that only you can have.

To produce flow experiences, however, depends on how you self-regulate thought processes in response to high-stress workout environments. If you are focused on keeping up with the person next to you, you may produce more internal stress (anxiety), which can negatively affect your behavior and diminish your workout. Or you can attempt to change your "construal" of the environment by focusing on yourself and just *exercising well,* which can positively affect your behavior and enhance your workout, and not obsessing about what is going around you so that it prompts a different and unfavorable behavior. Producing flow experiences means to focus on yourself and exercising well. Start by focusing on enjoying the exercise experience.

The concept of 'flow' is characterized by an "intense and focused concentration on what one is doing in the present moment" unimpeded by contrary pleasures, which only reduce the flow.[46] Flow experiences are described as being fully immersed in a *goal-directed activity* requiring the investment of "psychic energy" and is intrinsically rewarding after overcoming the challenge.[47] Flow, in the context of exercising, is a skill in acquiring a razor-sharp single-point unhindered concentration by focusing on the movement of a limb on the body in every stride, revolution, step, rep and set in an instant of time. It is training at an optimal level and enjoying the experience at the same time in that moment.

A distinctive feature of optimal experience that takes place is people become so involved in what they are doing that the activity becomes spontaneous, almost automatic; they stop being aware of themselves as separate from the actions they are performing and sense that they have become one with the activity itself.[48]

The feeling of flow can be described during a set of reps in weight training: "Your concentration is complete – one with the activity, one with the machine, and how it is making your body feel and challenging your mind. You feel the burn but the endorphins have kicked in. Your mind doesn't wander. If the mind wanders, the exercise becomes harder, more unbearable because your focus is elsewhere. You are not thinking of something else; you are totally involved with what you are doing and nothing else. The burning sensation subsides and you challenge yourself to keep going. You are strong and your energy is flowing. You feel relaxed, comfortable and energetic all at the same time."

Flow might be described as encompassing many flow experiences continuously training at peak level: "Your mind-body connection is strong-willed that by the snap your fingers you can smash workouts! It's the *tenacity* of repeating workout routines over and over until the *mind* becomes stronger and self-absorbed by the stimuli in the present movement of the activity and *wills* a higher level of training and removes *unwanted* contrary pleasures outside of itself that only negate subsequent peak level performances."

An optimal "flow" experience describes a sense of seemingly effortless movement, but it is far from being so. It requires strenuous physical exertion and disciplined mental activity. Any lapse in concentration will erase the "flow."[49] The purpose of the flow is to keep it going. It is not a constant upward motion, but rather a constant flowing stream of motion like the current of a river that occasionally changes yet keeps flowing.

If the flow lapses by focusing on a goal that is outside of itself, like beating an opponent, trying to impress someone or trying to make a lifting PR, then *competition* is likely to be a distraction to having a flow experience, rather than an incentive to focus on what is happening right now and have an optimal training experience.[50]

Suppose you fail to have a flow experience because your mind was focused on trying to make a lifting PR and got you anxious. Your thought processes prompt you to evaluate the failure and your focus is re-directed to stimulate a flow experience. You do another exercise and try a technique that is fresh and spontaneous to initiate the flow. And it works! Exercise flow experiences happen by engaging in an activity for its own sake that is self-directed. The reward is intrinsic, which can make struggling enjoyable and often discovering hidden opportunities for making progress.[51]

Ordering of Rules for the Flow

Rules of an activity help to keep the flow moving. Weight training, like other activities, has rules that require the learning of skills to exercise well in order to meet goals and provides self-evaluative feedback.[52] The various methods and systems of weight training along with its variables of sets, reps, rests and when, what and how much to eat are designed to make weight training an optimal exercise experience to achieve a goal. These rules also include an "ordered pace" of exercising (i.e., the amount of rest time between sets or none at all) in order to keep the flow of the body in motion to achieve muscle tension and reach the desired results in a reasonable amount of time.

The reason why flow improves the quality of experience is because its structured activity imposes order and excludes the "interference of disorder" outside of it. Any activity that requires concentration has a narrow window of time. A temporal focus is the only thing that counts. All the troubling thoughts (outside the activity) that ordinarily keep passing though the mind is temporarily kept in abeyance.[53]

For a basketball player the court is the only thing that matters. For a dancer the dance studio is the only thing that matters. For a bodybuilder the gym is the only thing that matters. For a soccer player the field is the only thing that matters. For the tennis player the court is the only thing that matters.

Enjoyable activities require a complete focusing of attention on the task at hand. The task at hand for a basketball player is to assist the team in making baskets and win the game. The task at hand for a dancer is to move the body in a rhythmic and energizing way and take delight in the movement. The task at hand for a bodybuilder is to train for constant tension and the pump for muscle growth. The task at hand for a soccer player is to assist the team in making goals and win the game. The task at hand for a tennis player is to make the ball go over the net and keep it away from his opponent to win points.

How a Flow Experience Begins

Here's how a flow experience begins. Start by zeroing in on an activity of an exercise for 30 seconds, such as biking, walking, running, bicep curls, squatting, etc. Feel the energy flowing from the limbs you are moving and the muscles you are exercising. See yourself occupying a single point in space. Nothing else matters around you. Freeze this space like a "snapshot." You are dynamic in this space. Do another 30 seconds, and so on.

Immerse yourself in what you are doing in that dynamic instant of time, in that moment. For instance, if you are on the stairmill, then focus on each deliberate step you take with *each leg*. If you are on the treadmill, then focus on each deliberate stride you take with each leg. If you are on the bike, then focus on each forceful rhythmic revolution you make with each leg. For example, if your goal is to cycle one mile in 3 minutes, then focus on the flow of each revolution of your legs while monitoring the distance covered every 30 seconds and each minute.

And if you are doing the battle ropes, the rope trainer, tubes, dumbbells, or the arm cranker for upper body strength and conditioning, then focus on each push or pull of *each arm* using the chest, triceps, shoulders, lats, and biceps. The challenge of flow experiences is rewarding because they are met with maximizing the exercise effort *in* that experience 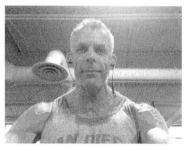 right then, right now. And where there is focus, effort invariably follows.

Building up the skill of flow experiences enables you to focus *in* the moment, in that instant of time, and work your muscles deliberately with a kind of mental energy you never knew you had.

Flow experiences help you focus on what you are doing *in* an activity of an exercise (what is happening now) rather than focusing on completing the whole activity (the long duration), which can hinder the flow and zap your energy making what feels to be an imaginative long and painful *exercise session* to complete.

Flow experiences enable you to discover yourself, to be yourself because its sole purpose is to optimize a training experience – your experience. And only you can experience your own, that is, if you are selfish in your pursuit to gain advantage to have a stronger and fitter body for yourself.

Practicing a Flow Experience

The time is now. Put your cell phones away. There is no texting and no selfie's during your flow experience. You are at the gym to work on you and focus on what you are doing now. You are a work in progress. Pause for a moment before you warm-up. Size up your surroundings. Now find your space in your present moment. Ready yourself for a flow experience and subsequent others. Get your head into the game. It is your time. Be first-rate to train at an optimal level. Turn up the music and let's go!

Concentrate. Zone in. Tune into your body. Connect your mind to your body. Don't let your mind wander. Every time you look at others in the gym your energy gets zapped. Focus on you; your every flow in every motion, every second, every minute. Freeze your space and focus in at the present moment. Immerse yourself in each dynamic instant of time. Reach into your mental energy. Train hard. Push yourself.

Don't let up. Pain is temporary. Suffer through it. There's light at the end of the tunnel. Look! You've become so focused in on the movement of the exercise that you hit a runner's high.[54] You no longer feel pain. You are unreceptive to it because of the release of natural occurring endorphins in your body to block the pain. You keep driving through effortlessly because you are in a state of euphoria. You did it! You had a flow experience and overcame yourself. Congratulate yourself. That's one day. Tomorrow is a new day.

Prepare yourself to have flow experiences every workout so you can overcome yourself every day to succeed. Mastering flow experiences will enable you to train continuously for 30 seconds, then 60 seconds, 2 minutes, 5 minutes, 10 minutes, and finally 60 minutes – unhindered by contrary pleasures and in harmony with your thoughts and feelings.

Visualization to Enhance a Flow Experience

Bodybuilders have said that the most productive workouts first begin in the head hours before the actual workout takes place. It is important to mentally rehearse your workout at least an hour before arriving to the gym.

Before you begin your workout sit down for a few moments and think about what you will do and how you will feel. Imagine yourself overcoming a hard workout. Do not rush to the gym after work because of an appointment you might have after your training session. Let your mind get in touch with your body and muscles.

When you are working out use a process called visualization. Visualization can help you concentrate on the movement of the exercise that you are performing and enhance flow experiences. It is forming a mental picture of yourself and visualizing what you must do to be a first-rate exerciser. I first learned about visualization in magazine articles from bodybuilders in the late 70s.

Arnold Schwarzenegger used visualization when he trained his biceps. He said he thought of his biceps as mountains, instead of flesh and blood. He claims that visualizing his biceps as mountains is what made his arms 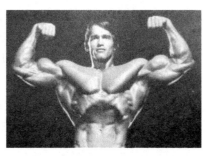 grow faster and bigger than if he'd seen them only as muscles. You may not have biceps like Arnold, but you can probably think of your biceps as hills developing *into* mountains with each peak contraction you do.

When you are doing chest flys visualize the movement like you are hugging a big tree. Visualize whatever can help you to stay focused on the task and make a mind-body connection. When you are doing lat pulldowns visualize your fingers as hooks so you only use your lat muscles to pull down the bar (to minimize your shoulders, traps, biceps and forearms), and then jab your elbows to your sides to contract or flex the lat muscles.

If you are spiritual, then get in touch with your "spiritual" side (the mind) when pushing or pulling against "matter" (the weights). Think of your lifting as a struggle between spirit and matter. Visualize spirit winning the battle over matter. Your mind is spirit and, therefore, good. The weight is matter and, therefore, evil. Matter is trying to crush you. Matter makes you weaker. Overcome matter with your mind to make you stronger.

You can use visualization when you are doing cardio. Take, for example, an upright bike. First, start peddling and set a resistance level that is challenging to cycle 3 miles in less than 10 minutes at 15-20 mph for a constant steady-state of 80-85%. Next, zone out of the gym and zone in on you. Connect your mind to your cardio objective.

Imagine that you are racing against elite cyclists in the Tour de France. By comparison their reality is a grueling, sweaty, rainy, bloody 2,156-mile stretch while yours is only 3 miles. Turn up your music and let the race begin! Find your cycle rhythm quickly to attain your speed and don't deviate from it but keep flowing with it. You are alongside elite cyclists racing for the prize! The mind-body connection becomes stronger with the flow and the constancy of the effort.

Flow Experiences 60 Minutes in a Day

To sustain a flow experience for 30-60 minutes not only requires consistency, but the *constancy of the effort* continually. In other words, staying on the path to the goal that holds a strong intrinsic value to you means more than sticking to a routine and exercising consistently day in and day out. It demands the constancy of the same or approximate level of intensity continually each and every day.

Exercising is a long-term commitment because you will never stop moving until you are dead. We must keep moving because our bodies are slowly deteriorating each year. Weight resistance training keeps the mind and body strong and energized and enduring in an electropositive charged condition.

Constancy Builds Small Empowering Habits

Constancy is about building small empowering habits and rituals that you partake in every single day that keep you focused on your highest priorities and goals. It essentially comes down to your ability to hold yourself accountable for the daily choices you make with no excuses and no complaints. You and you alone are accountable for what you do and what you fail to do.

Constancy is Focusing on the Instant

Constancy means to focus on the instant rather than the end goal. A flow experience allows you to zone in on what you need to get done before you zone in on another thing. It is an unrelenting focus. This is powerful because you can master one thing at a time in order to become very good at it. Focusing on one thing at a time repeatedly increases your efficiency and performance for what you want to produce or accomplish.

Multitasking does just the opposite. Several studies show that when you multitask your attention is diverted from one part of the prefrontal cortex of your brain to the other part. That takes time and reduces the quality of work.

Focusing on what you are doing now increases the efficiency of both parts of the brain working together and helps keep your attention on a single goal to carry out a specific task.[55] A good but crude example of experiencing the spontaneity of flow with an unrelenting focus to accomplish a specific task is the character John Wick.

HABIT #2

Experience the Flow of Exercising to Perform at an Optimal Level

CHAPTER 3

PHYSIOLOGICAL EFFECTS

Recuperation is your body's ability to recover *after exercise stress to increase functional performance and effect change.*[56]

Sufficient recuperation after a workout increases functional performance and effects body composition. Faster recovery means more strength and muscle and fat loss quicker in a shorter amount of time. Building strength and muscle and losing fat occur during rest periods, after exercise – outside of the gym.

How Much and What Kind of Rest?

How much rest you require depends on six factors: (1) how *fast* your body recovers (recuperation); (2) how *hard* you exercise (intensity); (3) how *often* you exercise per week (frequency); (4) how *often, much, what* and *when* you eat (nutrition); (5) how *long* you exercise (duration); and (6) how *much* stress you have or are able to manage in your daily life (stress).

What kind of rest can include: (1) nightly REM sleep, (2) 15-minute power-naps, (3) cycling your training intensity,[57] (4) taking work or exercise days off, (5) involving yourself with an expressive hobby or (6) engaging in meaningful conversation.

Three Phases of Recuperation

Recuperation is the time it takes the body to recover from an exercise session. Increases in energy, strength, performance, and endurance can slow down or come to a screeching halt should you overlook the recuperation process. Recuperation is broken down into three phases: (1) 30 to 90 second rests between sets during exercise, (2) 30-minutes to 3 hours immediately after exercise, and (3) 48 to 72 hours after exercise.[58]

30-Minute Post-Exercise Nutrition

You are sweaty and exhausted after a 60 to 90-minute workout. What does the body need for recovery: protein or carbohydrates? Does the body need protein to repair muscles first? Or does the body need carbohydrates to replenish lost fluids first?

Sports nutritionist, Nancy Clark, says your top priority after a workout is to replace fluids lost from sweating so your body can get back into a water balance.[59] Simple carbohydrate fluid replacers like juices and fruit are the best "fast-acting" electrolyte sources. Eight ounces of orange juice seems to be the best fluid replacer because it contains more potassium than a medium banana and it is moderate-to-high on the glycemic index providing the quickest replenishment for *immediate* recovery.[60]

But this doesn't mean to avoid protein for recovery. If your meals are spaced out every 3 hours you should have an adequate amount of protein in your muscles on a daily basis to avoid muscle breakdown immediately after an exhausting workout.

However, your second priority is to consume a liquid or solid form of protein 30 to 45 minutes after your workout – ideally with carbohydrates. But you don't need a lot of protein. That is the myth. An adequate amount of protein can replace lost glycogen to restore energy in the body and promote muscle recovery.[61]

Interestingly enough, it has been shown in many studies with athletes that drinking chocolate milk offers a good balance of protein with carbohydrates.[62] It is not my choice of consumption (yet) but it appears to be an effective post-exercise choice because sugar is what the body needs to replace glycogen stores. However, it may not be a safe choice for someone who is lactose intolerant.

Carbohydrates and protein are a winning combination because both stimulate the action of insulin that transports glucose (glycogen) from the blood to the muscles that need repair.

Sports nutrition sources recommend a 3:1 ratio of carbohydrates to protein for immediate post-exercise nutrition recovery.[63] But it doesn't stop there. As part of the second phase of recovery, it is important to eat a complex carbohydrate and protein meal 60 to 90 minutes after a workout for *sustained* recovery.

Three Reasons for Recuperation

There are three main reasons why the body needs rest: (1) neurological, (2) physiological, and (3) psychological. The first reason allows the nervous system to recuperate (neurological).

When a person lifts weight for the first time, observe that the bar wavers, shakes and wobbles. The weight is all over the place except for where it should go. That is neurological. The body first learns how to lift a weight with the nervous system and sends signals to the brain to excite the muscles. Beginners notice considerable increases in strength. This is due to a neurological adaptation, not necessarily more muscle.

Not many training methods, as far I know, can overload the CNS, except for one that I have experienced. I used it at the turn of the millennium. It is called *Power Factor Training* (PFT).

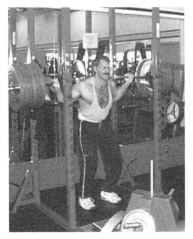

The idea behind PFT is to perform multiple strong-range partial reps with a lot of weight. According to PFT, strength and muscle "gains" are calculated by a mathematical computation called the Power Factor Index (PFI).

The PFI is calculated by multiplying the amount of weight used in an exercise by how many reps are performed, and dividing the result by the duration of the exercise in minutes. For example, performing 15 partial rep squats with 600 pounds in 1 minute the PFI would be 9,000 per minute.

Determining the PFI for the duration of the workout is the same except the number is reduced by moving the decimal over once to the left for the convenience of tracking a lesser number. Let's say, for example, 100,000 pounds was lifted in 60 minutes. The PFI for the workout would not be 1,666 but rather 167.

The whole idea with PFT is to lift as much weight as you can in as many strong-range partial reps as you can in the shortest amount of time for the duration of the workout. More weight lifted in less time means a higher PFI and, thus, a purported increase in strength and muscle.

The author of PFT claims that the PFI is a measurement of muscular output. However, the biggest problem with this is that the measurement doesn't take into account *the distance* the weight is lifted, which determines the actual amount of muscular output performed. Thus, PFI is not a measurement of power.

I stopped PFT after 6 weeks because my CNS was rundown from overexerting every ounce of brain power, muscle fibers and nerves within my ectomorphic build to lift excessive poundage's multiple times.

Fortunately, I walked away injury free. PFT did not benefit my body. When I went back to my regular training performing full-range reps my strength and body composition remained the same.

The only thing that PFT gave me was a huge ego-trip making me believe I was lifting "thousands" of pounds and getting stronger when I wasn't. I failed to take into account leverage factors and the distance of the weight lifted. The bottom line is that full-range movements stimulate more muscle fibers resulting in a higher work output:

Greater Distance → Increased Fiber Stimulation →
Higher Work Output = More Muscle

The second reason why the body needs rest is to permit sufficient "supercompensation" to take place (physiological). This is when the whole body has the opportunity to become stronger and more efficient. Supercompensation is discussed more in detail below. Not only does each muscle exercised need rest, i.e., "specific rest", but the whole body needs rest in order to regenerate itself, i.e., "general rest." If the whole body is excluded to rest, then too much stress can build up and can steer the body into an "over-trained" state.

Overtraining is produced by excesses in three main areas: volume, frequency, and intensity. Few people train too hard. Instead, most train too much and too often. An over-trained state is not pleasant. Watch out for these warning signals: (1) lack of motivation, (2) loss of strength, (3) loss of weight, (4) sickness, etc. A lack of rest can interrupt and slow down the body's recuperative ability. Giving the body complete rest is necessary to renew it with energy and vigor and allow stress to dissipate. Overtraining is discussed more in Chapter 6.

The third and last reason why the body needs rest is to sustain motivation (psychological). Becoming discouraged by not having the get-up-and-go kind of motivation and enjoy training hard can be largely due to a lack of rest for both the mind and the body. This can lead to a psychological "burn-out" and might make you want to take a hiatus from training longer than you wish.

The "Intensity" Factor

Rest time depends on how hard or intense you train. Intensity is not about how much you can lift, but *how well* you can stimulate the muscles for each rep of every set given the amount of "time under tension." Training hard means more rest is necessary for the body to recover. Retired 6-time Mr. Olympia Dorian Yates only trained four times a week due to his one all out set of an exercise of high-intensity training (HIT).

Rarely a beginner is too intense because he is still learning the motion and how to exercise. You cannot run first before you can walk. It's all about coordination and muscular contraction. Most beginners cannot grasp the intensity of advanced trainees because they lack the know-how and experience. Like anything else, intensity is a learning process. I talk more about intensity in Chapter 5.

Do Your Homework Outside the Gym

Time out! Your first priority outside the gym is to provide adequate high-performance nutrition between workouts and enough rest time to allow proper and sufficient recovery to take place. If you wish to reap the rewards from hard training to incinerate fat and build muscle, then nutrition and rest are inseparable. If the allotted recovery time and performance nutrition is ignored, then it is of little consequence. Physiological changes occur between workouts, but only if provided enough time and the proper nutrition to produce what is called the "Supercompensation Effect."

Time out! Each one of us has a unique recovery time due to our body's response to post-exercise stress and how efficient our body absorbs nutrition. Keep in mind that an extra day or two of rest is more beneficial to the body than another day of training. Be honest with yourself. In this case, don't listen to your mind; listen to your body. If you are exhausted one day or in doubt of your recovery time, then take a day off.

The Supercompensation Effect

Supercompensation simply refers to your body's recuperative ability to recover after exercise. See the diagram below with the corresponding numbers in parenthesis. Supercompensation constitutes three phases: recuperation (3), restoration (5), and supercompensation (6). It is based on a combination of smart and hard training with performance nutrition and sufficient recovery time.

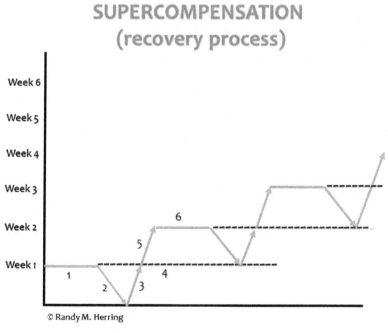

SUPERCOMPENSATION
(recovery process)

© Randy M. Herring

Post-exercise stress

The *right amount of exercise stress* applied to training (1) results in the breakdown and damage of muscle fibers, which places the body in a weakened and vulnerable state (2). This damage manifests itself as muscle soreness. During the recuperative phase (3), the damaged muscle fibers are rebuilt or restored and made stronger than they were before from the previous workout (4) in order to meet the increased stress demand of future workouts (5), thereby allowing Supercompensation (6) to take place.

Understanding Supercompensation is important because it gives hindsight into *how* to lose weight and build muscle. Once again, and to repeat in another way, after a workout your body's priority is to recover from the systematic stress and fatigue incurred from training (1). The body's repair mechanism kicks into effect, a process which, if given sufficient time (3) makes the damaged muscle fibers (2) thicker and stronger (5) than they were before from the previous workout (4). Due to hard training (1) coupled with performance nutrition and sufficient rest (3), the damaged muscle fibers (2) surrender to a new level of strength and growth (5), and, as the result, they supercompensate (6).

HABIT #3

Recover Sufficiently After Post-Exercise Stress to Effect Change

CHAPTER 4

PSYCHOLOGICAL VALUATIONS

Acquire an athletic mindset to train first-rate anywhere and anyhow and make exercising more precise and exacting.

Aristotle did everything under the sun. Primarily a scholar and philosopher in the community, his writings embody a wide range of areas seeking to understand our world and how to live well: psychology, biology, ethics, meteorology, physics, poetry, politics, metaphysics, logic, rhetoric, and other areas of interest. He was also a husband and father.

Aristotle's primary aim in the *Ethics* is to teach us how to become good human beings and attain happiness. Since that is our goal, we must demonstrate moderation in all things and be guided by "the golden mean."

Three Types of Mindsets

The golden mean is taking the right course of action in response to circumstances. Aristotle first distinguishes between three dispositions or states of character. Each disposition is inclined to take a certain course of action, which, in the case below, is in the sphere of fear and confidence.[64] I have called these dispositions mindsets. One mindset is the mean between two extreme mindsets; one is excess of the right course of action and the other deficiency.

Because two mindsets are extreme, they are undesirable. The mindset in the middle is good and desirable because it takes the right course of action for "what the circumstances demand."[65] Each "X" indicate that the right course of action under extreme circumstances could involve being near the middle but leaning toward one extreme than the other. But the middle, the mean, is what is moderate for the right course of action.

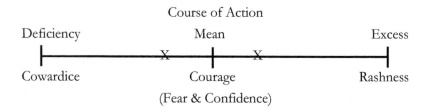

The middle is described as "courage" because it produces a mean. It deals with bravery involving two feelings: confidence and fear. These two feelings lie between the two extremes. To act rashly is to have too much confidence in excess of courage. To act cowardly is to have too much fear in deficiency of courage. Excess and deficiency are contrary to the right course of action. What all this means is that it is difficult business to become a good human being because *not* everyone can be moderate and take the right course of action in all circumstances and *hit the target* at the center of a circle.

In other words, it is easy to be disposed toward a certain feeling (like fear or confidence), but it is difficult to act towards the *right person* to the *right extent* at the *right time* for the *right reason* in the *right way,* and therefore, hit the target in the middle to take the right course of action to become a good human being.

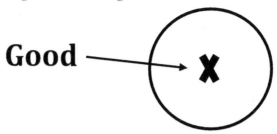

Good

To become a good human being is essentially to become all things to all human beings. And this is a difficult task. But if we are to attain our goal, we must suffer through it like an athlete in training. We must do our best to come close to hitting the middle of the target to obtain the desired goal, the prize.[66]

Aristotle's golden mean can be our guide when we are faced with a challenging or threatening situation. We can choose to fight to overcome it by either being brave and act at the mean with courage (Aristotle) or being a bit over the top and act toward the excess from the mean as a "warrior" (Nietzsche). Either fighting response puts us in touch with our sympathetic nervous system and allows us to use the adrenaline and fight harder.[67] When we fight that which threatens us, we affirm ourselves and the suffering itself which belongs to life and it strengthens us.[68]

Suffering through something and overcoming it makes us a better and stronger person. We suffer *through* self-discovery. We suffer *through* decision-making. We suffer *through* right-acting. We suffer *through* right-belief. We suffer *through* training. Why do we want to suffer through all of this? We do it for the self-satisfaction for desiring to take hold of *a value for which we fight.*

What does all this Aristotelian right acting and Nietzschean suffering have to do with exercise, and specifically applying it to weight resistance training? The parallel is this: It may be easy to "lift weights," but it is difficult to *train* for the results you desire with the *right routine,* the *right amount of intensity,* the *right form,* and eat the *right foods* in the *right amounts* at the *right time* and *often enough,* and have the *right attitude* toward your desired goal and suffer through it to attain it.

Hitting the target with the right amount of everything in your training and suffering through it with an athletic mindset makes exercising more precise and exacting.

The Great Health

An athletic mindset stems from well-disposed habits that can give birth to what Nietzsche calls *the great health.*[69] It is a new robust health, stronger, more seasoned, tougher, more audacious, and happier than any previous health. It is a great health that one "acquires continually" from the adventures of his or her own "authentic experience" that is yet undiscovered overflowing with power and abundance.

Valuation Excuses

What is your excuse for not trying to discover your great health? What is your excuse for not being a cause to accomplish your design? What is your excuse for not exercising? What is your excuse for not acquiring the mindset to accomplish these?

I can't...because I don't have time. I can't...because I'm too busy. I can't...because I have a fast metabolism. I can't...because I have the fat gene. I can't...because I have issues. I can't...because I am missing a limb. I can't...because I have injuries. I can't...because I have low testosterone. I can't...because I am too old. I can't...because I don't have good genetics. I can't...because I don't have the proper exercise attire. I can't...because I have limited exercise equipment. I can't...because gyms are expensive to join. I can't...because gyms intimidate me. I can't...because my gym isn't a positive environment. I can't…because of COVID-19. I can't…because of lockdown. I can't…because I have to wear a face mask exercising.[70]

All these are *valuation excuses* we talk ourselves into believing. Such beliefs make us accept our own closures and limit our possibilities. We tend not to believe in ourselves when we either compare ourselves with others or are faced with obstacles. Is it because we feel like we can't measure up to others or overcome our own excuses? Who's to blame? I AM…because it is MY mindset.

My First Transformation

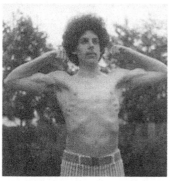

At 15-years-old I weighed a mere 115 pounds. I wanted to gain weight because I was skinny and bullied. I was too intimated to join my local gym so I trained at home with a barbell and dumbbell set doing basic exercises and with no nutritional guidance for six months from December to June.

I lifted weights every day three times a day because I thought I had to train a lot to build muscle. I was wrong! After 6 months, I only put on 10 pounds. At 125 pounds I was still skinny for two reasons. One, I didn't eat enough food. And two, I exercised too much.

In June I invested in a weight gain diet mail order by Universal Bodybuilding. It was high in protein, carbs and fat. I worked as a dishwasher for a local restaurant so I had a burger with fries or French dip and a slice of cherry pie during my breaks.

I followed this weight gain diet for 8 months. I ate six meals daily, which were evenly spaced out about 3 hours. I got up at 6am to eat my first meal and went back to bed before getting up 3 hours later for my next meal. I ate meat and cheese, gorged on desserts, drank lots of milk, ate a lot of bread and consumed nightly protein drinks.

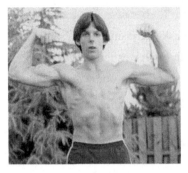

In February, and eight months later, I tipped the scales at 180 pounds. My waistline ballooned from 27 to 36 inches. I was fat but felt confident about myself because I transformed the skinny kid that I once was into a more confident and stronger kid. Shortly thereafter, I invested in another diet and training program mail order to lean out.

This program was from none other than the Austrian Oak, the greatest, the one and only, the king himself, my idol, Arnold Schwarzenegger. I lost 25 pounds in four months.

At 155 pounds I was stronger, more confident and had a better physique. In my first year of serious training and investing in two training and nutrition plans I gained 30 pounds of lean muscle training at home. I joined a local athletic club three months later. I met Arnold Schwarzenegger the same year that summer.

Arnold Schwarzenegger

Meeting Arnold Schwarzenegger is life-changing. He was in Portland, Oregon doing a book signing for his autobiography, *Arnold: The Education of a Bodybuilder.*

I was in awe of his presence. My hero. My idol. Six-time Mr. Olympia. The icon of *Pumping Iron.* The greatest physique of all time.

I nervously approached him and handed him my book to sign. I said, "hi." He said, "hi." Wow! We exchanged a few words! I was too nervous to talk to him. But I can say we almost had a conversation.

A year after I met Arnold, I graduated from high school. I moved into an apartment in my hometown. I am 17.

Train First-Rate

While living by myself and training at the local gym I wrote a letter to Arnold. I asked him about my belief of moving to Venice Beach, California to train at the famous Gold's Gym where "positive thinking" is contagious. My head was in the clouds and I was possessed with a streak of idealism of becoming a world-class bodybuilding champion like himself.

Arnold responded to my somewhat boyish question in *Muscle & Fitness* magazine within a few months. His reply devastated me. He said, "If you can't be a first-rate bodybuilder where you are at, then forget it." I hated him and felt stupid for even asking the question. But as the years rolled by Arnold's answer made more sense to me. I thought: "I can train *first-rate* anywhere and feel like a first-rate bodybuilder."

In my mind, my excuse for not even trying to train first-rate was the perception that my geographical location and training environment was a disadvantage to me. In short, my excuse was psychological. It was my mindset. I had it set in my mind that my hometown and local gym was unacceptable because it did not match up to the famous Gold's Gym in Venice Beach, California – the Mecca of Bodybuilding.

Arnold's answer challenged a quest to acquire an athletic mindset to train first-rate at any gym from my hometown gym in Gresham, Oregon and Gold's Gym in Venice Beach to gyms across the country and overseas.

A year after graduating from high school and living on my own I had the opportunity to go to college in California. Before I quit my job and left my hometown, I ventured out into the wild to explore the Mount Hood Wilderness for a few days and to climb Mount Hood that summer.[71] I knew I would miss the Pacific Northwest (with the exception of the rain). I am 18.

The Mecca of Bodybuilding

I moved to California and stayed with my mom in Newport Beach for a month before college. But college wasn't on my mind. It was Gold's Gym. I was drawn towards it. My mindset was and always had been to train at the gym where champions are made. After all, it was now just a hop, skip and jump away!

I woke up one morning with the idea of riding my yellow 10-speed Schwinn bicycle along Pacific Coast Highway to Gold's Gym. After all, Venice Beach is on the coast. I reasoned that if I rode along Pacific Coast Highway I would eventually arrive at my destination.[72] My mom was at work and I didn't tell her what I was doing. So, I set out on my journey without a map. And Google Maps wouldn't be available until the turn of the millennium.

Twenty miles and an hour and a half into my bike ride I got two flat tires. I rode my bicycle over gravel embedded with thorns. It was hot and I coughing because I was in a smog-infested industrial area. I walked my bike over to a nearby café and asked the waitress where I was. She said Long Beach. I discovered that I had three more hours and 33 miles to go – not even half-way to Gold's Gym.

I saw a pay phone outside the café. I put a quarter in the coin slot and called my mom. I told her of my whereabouts to pick me up. To this day, I do not know how she found me. When my mom arrived, she was very upset, but thankful that I was alright. I put my 10-speed in the back of her Porsche 924 and she raced home to get back to work.

Fitness in the Holy Land

Fast forward 10 months after my first year of college. I am working and living in the Holy Land during the summer. I am 19.

Ever since I caught the fitness bug, I have found creative ways to be physically active or at least challenge my physical and mental skills where a gym was inaccessible while living and working overseas.

I was chosen as one of thirty college students among 200 applicants from various private universities across the country to act in two Christian plays in the Holy Land. The Jerusalem Passion Play (JPP) was performed on the Mount of Olives in Jerusalem and The Nativity Play of Bethlehem (NPB) was performed in Shepherd's Field in Beit Sahur near Bethlehem. I was cast as the disciple Thaddeus in the former and a Roman soldier in the latter.

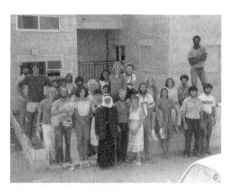

Every day was long arduous hard work from early morning until late evening. We, the JPP crew, were construction workers by day, rehearsing our roles by day, actors by night, security guards by day to morning and cooks at night. We lived in a three-story Jerusalem Stone house together.

Within a week after my arrival and adjusting to my new working life in Jerusalem, I adopted a basic training routine. I received *Muscle & Fitness* magazine issues from my mom every now and then to keep me motivated and my mind active. I also listened to my "Rocky" soundtrack cassette tape with my Walkman to keep me motivated in my workouts.

I exercised three times a week for 15 to 30-minutes. I did push-ups, ab crunches, leg raises, jumped rope, ran in place, ran around the block a couple of times in my neighborhood and finished with isotension training by flexing a muscle and holding the contraction.

After two and a half weeks, I started to be more creative with my training. One day I found a 30-pound log outside our house. I used the log primarily for shoulder flexibility and did presses behind the neck. I also started doing hack squats and isotension calf raises.

After nearly three weeks my training routine developed into this:

1. Crunches 2 x 60
2. Lying leg raises 2 x 50
3. Twists 2 x 60
4. Jump rope 2-4 minutes
5. Hack squats 3 x 30
6. Calf raises 3 x 12 (isotension 20 seconds for each rep)
7. Wide push-ups 5 x 15 (isotension for chest)
8. Press behind neck with 30-pound log 5 x 20
9. Narrow push-ups 5 x 10 (isotension for triceps)

The fourth week I jogged from the house to the Old City of Jerusalem and back. My goal was to do it in one hour and I did. A few days after this, and after a 30-minute workout in the morning, I jogged across the Judean desert to Shepherd's Field from the house. The house was located on the outskirts of Jerusalem and near a road heading to Bethlehem. My goal was to reach Shepherd's Field in one hour and I did.

I took a picture of the Judean desert in the direction that I would jog. "Aim straight and over the hills to Shepherd's Field," I said to myself. I jogged and walked up and down hills in the hot desert. I saw a few caves and always feared of running into rattlesnakes or scorpions. Fortunately, that never happened.

Shortly arriving at Shepherd's Field, I told the director what I did. He exclaimed, "You did what!? You're crazy!"

Five days after jogging across the Judean desert I jogged from the Mount of Olives to the house. I arrived at the house in an hour and a half soaked in sweat. One of the actors exclaimed, "You're out of your mind!" Five minutes after I arrived, I had a 45-minute workout.

In mid-August a few of us JPP actors were cast as extras in an American film that was being shot in Jerusalem called *Remembrance of Love,* a story about Holocaust survivors. The movie stars Kirk Douglas and Pam Dawber. I played 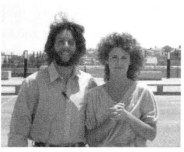 a cameraman. I got paid 250 shekels for my part in the movie.

This was my life and fitness lifestyle in the Holy Land. I did what I could and did what was challenging so that I could succeed and feel the self-satisfaction. I adapted to my overseas experience and the environment. Physical fitness is, after all, intrinsically rewarding for how it makes you feel. The inevitable reward is the physical results from the *process* of doing it.

Both play productions closed prematurely due to a lack of tourism. The war between Israel and Lebanon intensified when Israel invaded Lebanon the beginning of summer.

Fitness in Montana

I flew from Israel to New York to Missoula, Montana. I stayed with my grandmother until my second year of college would begin three weeks later. The day after I arrived in Missoula, I began looking for a gym. I found one called Wallwork's Gym. After settling into my new surroundings, I had my first workout three days later.

I jogged to Wallwork's Gym one afternoon for my first workout. I did abs, calves, chest, shoulders and arms for an hour. After the workout I walked home and I was thinking that I only had two and a half weeks before returning to school. That meant that I had 16 days to smash my workouts! I pulled myself together and focused on eating better and having hard consistent workouts. I wrote down everything I ate and paid special attention to my calorie and carbohydrate numbers.

The next day I jogged to the gym for my second workout. I did abs, calves, quads, hams, traps and forearms for an hour and a half. It was an intense workout because I almost threw up.

After these first two workouts and on the sixth day after arriving in Missoula, I wrote down a training schedule plan for 16 days. I followed a 3-day a week split routine where I trained each muscle group once every two to three days a week, and trained abs and calves every day. Day 1: chest, shoulders and triceps; Day 2: legs, back, traps, biceps and forearms; Day 3: deadlifts; Day 4: repeat. I rotated the order of some exercises and substituted some exercises for others.

I also wrote down a daily training plan of what exercises I would do for each muscle group before I got to the gym so that I didn't leave myself hanging wondering what I would do.

The next day, I was scheduled to do deadlifts. But not even halfway through my workout I terminated it. I was not mentally into it.

The following day in the early afternoon, to clear my head, I ventured out to hike up to the top of Mount Sentinel for the first time. I didn't take a path, but rather made my own path through the high brush and hiked straight up to the top.[73] Hiking Mount Sentinel would become a routine hike for me in the years ahead doing it three to four times a year in spring and summer.

After coming down from the mountain, I had a double-split training session in the late afternoon and mid-evening. I did legs for one session and back, traps, biceps and forearms for the other session. The following day I did the same. I did chest in the afternoon and shoulders and triceps in the evening. I did more sets per muscle group than what I was accustomed to and kept my reps at eight. The next day I revisited deadlifts.

Deadlifts: King of Exercises

I have always been good at doing high-volume deadlifts. I journaled my first deadlift workout a few weeks into my first year in college. Within a month, I was deadlifting over 300 pounds on a consistent basis for reps. A Samoan by the name of Tali exclaimed, "Iron Randy is back!"

I consider deadlifts the king of exercises. First, it is a functional exercise. Second, it can increase core strength, power, muscle and cardiorespiratory conditioning. And three, it can boost metabolism.

Before I actually did my first deadlift workout at Wallwork's I mentally rehearsed it before I got to the gym. I saw a clear picture of myself completing the last and hardest lift.

During my actual workout I did exactly what I mentally rehearsed in my head. I did four sets of 10 before doing my last set with 305 for 1 rep max (1RM). But I only had four more deadlift workouts to go before the day I turned 20. I wanted to give myself a personal record (PR) as a gift to myself on my birthday.

The next day, after a chest workout, I was looking through a *Muscle & Fitness* magazine issue. I was reading how bodybuilders made their workouts highly effective. Here are a few:

"...the head is the secret." – Lou Ferrigno

"I firmly believe in the old proverb, 'Whatever can be conceived and believed can be achieved." – Boyer Coe

"Mentally programming yourself for success and then letting your body follow through on that plan of action." – Laura Combes

"...develop a tremendous mental drive to carry you through many years of consistent hard training." – Franco Columbu

My second deadlift workout improved. I did the same first four sets with the same weight and reps. On my fifth and final set I did 305 for 3RM. That night I dreamed that I was preparing to deadlift 535 pounds. But in my dream, it was a failed attempt.

My third deadlift workout was mind-blowing. I increased the weight by 20 pounds for the first three sets of 10 reps. I increased the next set by 50 pounds for 6 reps. And I increased the fifth set to 325 and did 4 reps. I tried to pull 375 by yelling the weight up for 1RM but I failed.

My fourth deadlift workout was better than the previous one. I did seven sets. The first five sets were the same as the last workout. I attempted 375 again and yelled up a 2RM. On my seventh set I increased the weight to 425. I focused on a PR by channeling my mind and energies throughout my whole body. And I did it, but only by yelling the weight up. I had one more deadlift workout to go and I knew I could do better.

I am 20. Happy birthday to me. My fifth and last deadlift workout was a PR. I increased the weight by 30 pounds for the first three sets for 10 reps and also the fourth set for 6 reps. On my fifth set I increased the weight by 30 pounds for 4 reps. On my sixth set I added 50 pounds from my fifth set. I pulled 405 for 3RM on my twentieth birthday. That's a 100-pound increase in only three deadlift workouts in nine days!

I attempted 455 for a seventh set but failed. But I was able to reclaim it 24 years later at 44 for 5RM. As my body matured in my 40s, I was able to consistently pull 315 for 15 and 405 for 10.

After 16 days of intense and consistent training at Wallwork's Gym, I gained strength and muscle and lost fat. I weighed 168 pounds.

Meeting Bill Pearl

Fast forward six and a half years from California to Japan to graduating from college in California to Japan again and back to

Missoula in spring. I am working behind the front desk in a private gym in Missoula called The New Life Fitness Club.

One day a young athletic-looking lady approached the front desk to train as a guest. She told me she and her boyfriend and a couple of friend's trains with retired 4x Mr. Universe, Bodybuilding Hall of Fame and author of *Keys to the Inner Universe,* Bill Pearl at his home in Oregon.

The young lady's name was Jeanne. She gave me her work number and said if I was ever in the area to give her a call and she'll make arrangements so that I too could train with Bill Pearl. I was ecstatic!

I left Missoula in late August on route to southern California. I contacted Jeanne to let her know I would be in the area soon.

I arrived in Medford in the afternoon and checked into a hotel. I arranged to meet Jeanne and her boyfriend, Brad, outside my hotel early the next morning so I could follow them to Bill's ranch.

Excited and with little sleep, I was promptly up by 3:30 a.m. A two-hour workout with Bill begins at 4:00 a.m. sharp! I arrived at a barn with a fully furnished gym. I can confidently say with other athletes who have trained with Bill before dawn, "I survived the barn."

At the time, Bill was 58. And I was 26. Today he is 90 and I am 58. When I train myself these days, I sometimes reflect upon my observation of Bill's training back then and sense that he had a kind of methodical system of training. He trained not only with a sense of purpose but also with a keen sense of mind-body connection to make continual progress.

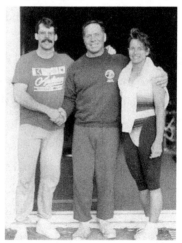

The mind-body connection, it seems, is a process that becomes engrained over the years by repetitive training habits with an approximate level of intensity to ensure a series of body transformations to keep the body strong and fit over the years. It's a kind of training that has been established by one's will that dictates a habitual behavioral pattern to keep fit-for-life.

Bill's training methodology is similar to my late grandmother's day-to-day routine. She had a good life and a heart of gold. She had a habitual routine that was simple, yet it kept her mind and body active. She got up every morning at the same time. She ate breakfast and read the newspaper. She ate a balanced lunch. She went for a walk outside when it was nice and took an occasional nap in the afternoon. She ate a hearty dinner before watching the news. She was an avid reader. Good healthy habits keep us strong and mindful. She lived to be 103. Like my grandmother, Bill is an inspiration. Dedication and commitment to a routine can help us live a long, mindful and healthy life.

After training, Bill and his wife Judy took us out for breakfast. I can't recall what we talked about. I can only recall that Bill was at the head of the table and I was sitting to his right. My conversation with Bill was surreal. When he looks and talks to you, he has this kind of intriguing sparkle in his eye and intense focus that he is truly interested in you.

After breakfast, I thanked Bill and Jeanne, got into my car and went back to my hotel. The next day I worked out at Superior Athletic Club before I left Medford. While driving through San Jose, California, I stopped off to workout at Gold's Gym. This is where I met the late bodybuilder, Scott Wilson.

After my workout at Gold's, I had a mind-altering moment. I turned around and headed north back to Portland. My dad was going through a difficult time and I felt that he needed my support at the time.

Fitness in Japan

I stayed with my dad for a couple of weeks until I had another mind-altering moment. I was moving to the Land of the Rising Sun. I sold my car and bought a one-way ticket to Japan. I packed my philosophy books, Brother typewriter, bowling ball, and dress clothes. I was in it for the long run: to teach, to study, to observe, to write, to travel and to exercise.

I had already lived and worked in Japan for two years on two separate occasions. I enjoyed teaching English conversation, the hospitable people and the hitch-hiking adventures.

I arrived in Japan early fall. I stayed at a friend's place in Tokyo for two weeks until I found work in Chiba. I moved to Chibadera, a suburb in Chiba, and lived in a modern one room apartment with a loft.

I bought a desk, chair, bookcases, futon and a kotatsu table heater. The next two months I focused on work, my students, and the company. I was working 20 hours a week and my living was comfortable. I had much leisure. I immersed myself in philosophy and wrote reflective essays. In the meantime, I needed to find a fitness center. But not having a gym available did not stop me from exercising.

I put together a 3-day a week full-body freehand exercise routine at home and did as many sets as it took to complete a predetermined rep range. I also discovered a track and field across the street from where I lived. I sprinted 100 meters on the straightaways to train my hamstrings and speed-walked the curves 100 meters for active recovery before sprinting the other straightaway and repeating. I did this eight times around the track to equal one mile.

When I finished my sprints, I did underhand pull-ups on a bar located above some bleachers. I did as many sets as it took to complete my rep range. I did this outside routine three times a week on alternate days from my full-body freehand routine at home. My routine looked like this:

Day 1: Home Routine
1. Elevated push-ups (upper chest) 50-100 reps
2. Push-ups (chest) 50-100 reps
3. Handstand push-ups (shoulders) 20 reps
4. Narrow hand push-ups (triceps) 60 reps
5. One or two-leg squats (quads) 80-400 reps
6. Elevated one-leg calf raises (calves) 60 reps

Day 2: Outside Routine
1. Straightway sprints (hams) 100 meters
2. Curve powerwalks (hams) 100 meters
   Repeat 8 more times
3. Underhanded pull-ups (back & biceps) 25-50 reps

There are many variations of positioning the body (feet elevated, piked position, knees on the floor, hands against the wall with feet out to modify resistance) when doing the home freehand routine, especially doing push-ups and handstand push-ups. It depends on your level of fitness, level of strength, and of course your own body weight, and injuries, if any.

A few months later, and the following year, I found a local community center in the city of Chiba that had a small gym and doable equipment. It had a universal weight machine, a bench press, a power rack and weights. This was all that I needed. It was hot and humid in the gym during summer because there were no windows or air conditioning.

To help myself with nutrition while in Japan my grandmother sent me a calorie counting book from the States that listed the amount of each macronutrient of a particular food. I also bought a nutrition "picture book" in Japan that listed certain foods that I ate so that I could see the item and help me know the serving size and amount of each macronutrient in roman numbers.

For my post-workout recovery, I frequently gulped down a liter of milk while walking down the street and ate a box of raisins on the train while heading to work. I frequently ate soybeans from a plastic bag on a train to feed my body at the proper times to promote muscle recovery after exercising.

In spring the following year, I discovered a newly built fitness center down the street from the community center called the Chiba Port Arena. It is a sports complex that hosts annual sporting events. The gym was small but larger than the community center and it was air 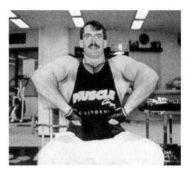 conditioned. The weight machines were new and modern and included the first "cardio" machines (e.g., treadmills) that I experienced.

I had to be creative with some exercises while working out at the Chiba Port Arena. The facility didn't have dipping bars. So, I performed dips between two treadmills using the handrails. It also didn't have an incline bench. I performed incline bench presses on an adjustable incline/decline ab bench. After I sat down on the floor and laid on the bench, I had two male staff workers give me the weighted bar and then take it from me when I completed each set.

I had a very fun, positive and unforgettable experience at both fitness centers because of the hospitable staff workers. The recession hit me hard, so in late spring I left Japan for the Middle East to be with my wife and first born. My second son was coming into the world in July.

Fitness in Beit Sahur

I lived in a beautiful two-story Jerusalem Stone house with my father and mother-in-law, my wife and first son.

The house was built on a higher foundation than street level. You had to open a gate under a stone entrance and walk up a few steps to the house. At the top of the steps, I used this overhead stone entrance to do pull-ups. I also did the freehand routine that I did in Japan in the house upstairs. I did push-ups elevated from the floor on three chairs by placing each palm and feet on each chair.

Within a week, I was working as co-owner of a local gym just down the street from the house. I worked there every day from open to close. Local fitness enthusiasts heard that an American was working there and made an effort to check out the gym.

The gym was dusty and dark and gloomy. Like the community center in Japan, this gym also had a universal weight machine. It also had a few benches, an Olympic bar, a pair of adjustable dumbbells and plates, but no air conditioning. And water was scarce. But the gym had everything necessary to promote physical fitness.

Early fall, and two months after my second son was born, my wife, myself and two boys left Beit Sahur for the States. We arrived in Michigan and stayed with my mom for two weeks. I financed a mini-van and traveled across the mid-west to Missoula. We stayed with my grandmother for two weeks until I found work in Spokane. We settled in Spokane Valley, Washington. I trained at a spacious and well-equipped fitness center that had a catchy name: *Sta-Fit.* I discovered it five years earlier passing through the area at the time that I met Bill Pearl.

Fitness Anywhere

Regardless what fitness centers or gyms look like, what the environment is like, and what kinds of equipment gyms have – all these things that we look for in a gym – it is important that you use what you have to your advantage and train first-rate, no matter how limited, how old fashioned or how different the equipment appears to be. If your exercise equipment is limited, then you have to work with what you have and be creative. It's perspective. It's mindset.

Basic compound exercises help increase strength, muscle and cardiorespiratory conditioning because they utilize a tremendous amount of energy in the body. There are many exercises that you can do at home with just a few plates, dumbbells, a chair, and body weight. The most inexpensive exercise equipment I ever purchased was a set of resistance exercise tubes with handles in anticipation of the first COVID-19 lockdown in spring 2020. Create opportunities to succeed rather than finding excuses that lead to failure without trying.

Acquire an Athletic Mindset

High-level peak performers are not addicted to work, they are addicted to results. Think about it. They have a mindset that is motivated by an intense drive towards success that manifests itself in a fierce single-pointed concentration. These peak efforts help *break through the mold* to higher functional levels. Peak efforts are powerful learning experiences and put us closer in touch with our "hidden reserves."

Quality of effort

Unleashing hidden reserves transmits itself into exerting a tremendous amount of effort that allows the body's adaptive mechanism to respond to many forms of exercise stimuli. There are no shortcuts to getting fit, getting stronger, learning how to do an exercise better, or producing great things in life. Acquiring wealth, learning skills, cultivating one or more of your intelligences takes time.[74]

The Greek philosopher, Democritus, wittingly says, "Learning achieves fine things through taking pains, but bad things one acquires without any pains."[75] Thus, fine things are not achieved without pain. Achieve fine things through taking pains by unlocking hidden reserves.

Work Miracles

In his essay *Self-Reliance*, Ralph Waldo Emerson writes, "Power is inborn. Throw yourself on this thought. Instantly right yourself. Stand in the erect position. Command your limbs. Work miracles."[76]

Habit #4

Acquire an Athletic Mindset to Train First-Rate Anywhere and Anyhow

CHAPTER 5

WEIGHT TRAINING AS THE EXERCISE MODALITY

Adopt a useful *low-impact exercise modality that is safe, fun and practical for the rest of your life.*

Enjoyment, low-impact, and good form go hand-in-hand if the goal is to exercise long-term, remain injury free and stay motivated.

My Second Transformation

My second transformation occurred 40 years later. I looked at myself in the mirror and felt disgusted. My pants were tighter, I didn't feel good about myself, and I wanted to feel and look better. I needed to change my lifestyle.

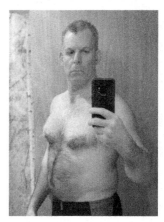

I increased my activity, changed my macronutrient ratio, prepped and ate six meals daily and stopped taking supplements and caffeine. I wanted to prove it to myself that I could make a total body transformation on my own by eating frequently throughout the day and training hard every day. I lost 17 pounds in the first 16 weeks and 25 pounds in one year.

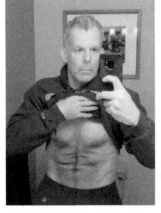

I exercised every day by rotating between a full-body weight training routine and a full-body cardio routine each performed 3-4 days a week. My weight routine consisted of high reps utilizing the reverse pyramid method. I incorporated supersets, burnsets, dropsets, rest/pause and partial reps in 60-minutes. I essentially trained for muscular endurance to burn fat, build muscle and increase endurance.

My cardio routine consisted of six cardio exercises for 10 minutes each training at a steady-state of 85% for 60-minutes. A high-intensity

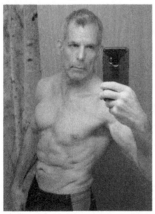

training (HIT) "steady-state" of at least 80% or higher for at least 45 minutes is superior to high-intensity interval training (HIIT) because it can give you more of an after-burn longer after exercise.

Training for muscular and cardiorespiratory endurance using both routines can make you feel better and see results within a week. They can also increase your physical fitness four-fold in 12 to 16 weeks. Each routine can incinerate up to 1,000 calories in 60 minutes.

Intensity (again)

Speed training, strength training, slow, deliberate and controlled muscle contractions, feeling your reps, counting your reps, high reps, low reps, five sets per exercise, three sets per exercise, heavy weight, moderate weight, light weight, etc.

Exercise training systems all tend to be confusing for increasing performance and improving appearance. Yet altering body composition and increasing fitness and functional ability remains the same and boils down to one word: intensity.

Unfortunately, the word intensity has many different meanings because the way in which it is defined and used according to a preferred exercise modality.

High-Impact Exercise Modalities

Before the word 'intensity' is defined let's first look at some general characteristics of functional training exercise modalities like CrossFit, Boot Camps and TRX. My intention is not to disapprove functional training exercise per se since experienced individuals or athletes can perform this modality well and enjoy it. My aim is directed toward those less experienced and less conditioned who might consider participating in group functional training sessions.

The first thing that these exercise modalities have in common is that you have to complete a certain number of exercises and reps as many times as possible in a limited amount of time.

For the most part, the idea is to perform a certain number of exercises (let's say five) in a sequential order for a certain number of sets and repetitions. For example, do as many burpees as you can in 8 minutes; perform squats, sit-ups, push-ups, rows, and burpees for 3 sets of 10 repetitions each with as much intensity as you can; do 3 sets of 12 front squats with a barbell, 10 pull-ups and 8 push presses as rapidly as possible; and finish up with a quarter-mile run.

The second thing that these exercise modalities have in common is the high-impact on the bones, joints and ligaments. People who have pre-existing injuries, joint issues and arthritis in the joints and wrist and fingers have difficulty performing these high-impact functional exercises safely.

Observation reveals that the majority cannot properly align their joints in a successful manner to do many of the exercises safely and effectively in regard to form in such a quick-paced workout. This can cause a lot of joint stress and subsequent joint issues and may put a halt to training either short or long-term in the desire to get fit.

Muscle Tension

High-intensity training (HIT) is a strength training system popularized in the 1970s by Arthur Jones. Repetitions are performed in a slow and controlled manner to the point of momentary muscular failure. The muscle is placed under "constant tension" during an amount of time it takes it to fatigue. This is especially true with eccentric training.

Eccentric training performed in a slow and controlled manner may have the upper hand in fatiguing the muscles quicker since this part of the motion focuses on the lengthening or elongation of the muscle, which can lead to stronger muscles faster.

The specific *time under tension* yields the greater amount of muscle stimulation at a given time and forces the muscle to fatigue and fail quick. The stress to the muscle causes it to adapt and get stronger after it recuperates, which stimulates growth.

You don't have to lift heavy to build muscle. Light weight and proper joint alignment with good form stimulates muscle growth. Focusing on each rep of a movement digs deep into the muscle and the painful "burning" sensation appears. You feel it because the brain tells you so.

The challenge, and the point, is to mentally remain in "the burn" (and not physically give up and terminate the set) doing full reps, then partial reps, and finally to controlled failure. The muscles have one option: adapt to the stress and re-build to get stronger and perform better next time (see the third habit and chapter on "recuperation" and the seventh habit and chapter on "adaptation").

Exercise intensity as it is applied to progressive weight resistance training can be defined as *the amount of force generated yielding the greatest number of muscle fibers stimulated at a given time.* Training hard (not necessarily "heavy") in the shortest amount of time (optimally) while stimulating the most muscle fibers is the ideal goal.

High-intensity training is seeking to make the muscles fail as quickly and effectively as possible. The process of high-intensity training that yields muscular growth follows this order: (1) proper joint alignment, (2) full range repetitions, (3) muscle isolation, (4) time under tension, (5) muscle failure, (6) muscle adaptation, and (7) muscle growth.

Measuring Cardio Exercise Intensity

Your heart is your most important muscle and your most vital organ. Knowing what your resting heart rate (RHR) is, is important because it can tell you a lot how fit or unfit you are. Calculating your target or training heart rate (THR) or target heart value (THV) will tell you how hard or easy your heart is working. This calculation is known as the *Karvonen Formula.*

Choose a heart rate technology that works best for you and one that is convenient to monitor your exercising heart rate. It's sort of like a personal trainer keeping you accountable to keep your heart rate in the desired range.

To know your THR you must first calculate *your* "theoretical" maximum heart rate (MHR). To calculate your MHR simply subtract your age from 220. This figure is your MHR. For example, 220 - 58 = 162. At my present age my MHR is 162.

Next, figure your RHR. It's best to take your RHR just after you become conscious in the morning. This is your "true resting heart rate."

Gently place your index and middle fingers over the wrist. You should feel a light pulsation. Count the number of beats for 6 seconds and multiply by 10. This will give you your RHR. A lower RHR means a stronger heart. It means that your heart is able to pump a higher volume of blood with one stroke throughout the body as opposed to taking two or three strokes for the same amount. Thus, a lower heart rate means more rests between beats and a stronger heart.

After that, subtract your RHR from your MHR. For example, 162 (MHR) - 55 (RHR) = 107. From this figure (107) multiply your desired exercise intensity. See the THR zone chart below. If I choose 76% (increase fitness) the figure will be 81 (107 x 76% = 81).

Finally, add your RHR to 81 (81 + 55 = 136). 136 would be a "low end" THR and 150 (107 x 89% = 95 + 55) would be the "high end" THR. I prefer to cardio train at a steady-state of 76-89% for an hour. I try to maintain the same THR intensity while bodybuilding-fitness training.

Training Heart Rate (THR) Zone

Effort	Percent of MHR	Objective	Fitness Level
1 to 3	0 to 59%	Moderate	Easy
4 to 6	60 to 75%	Weight Mgmt.	Endurance
7 to 8	76 to 89%	Increase Fitness	Endurance Edge
9 to 10	90 to 100%	Improve Performance	Elite

Resistance Exercise Tube Training

The first COVID-19 lockdown didn't stop me from training. When the State of Washington declared lockdown the beginning of spring and the State of Idaho followed 10 days later, my response to it was one of preparation. I bought a set of three resistance tubes with two handles two weeks earlier.

I had to adapt myself to the demanding circumstances to stay the course to continue making improvements to my body. Within a week, my "quarantine training" consisted of a full-body tube training routine similar to

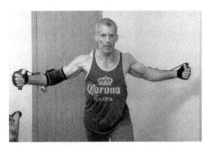

my gym routine. I also created a cardio tube routine for my upper body that consisted of 600-900 reps of 2-3 giant sets of six exercises for 25 reps each. I worked out every morning 7 days a week. The most difficult thing during this "test of time" was keeping my mind strong and disciplined.

Wall-Sits

Around this time, an acquaintance suggested wall-sits as an exercise to work the quads. I thought it was a silly suggestion. Boy, was I wrong! I began doing 3-minute wall-sits and in two weeks progressed to 5-minute wall-sits after my seventh wall-sit. In six weeks and after my fourteenth wall-sit I worked up to 7-minutes. My usual routine,

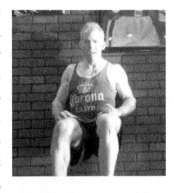

however, consisted of 4-minute wall-sits of 4-6 sets with 2-minute box steps intervals between each set for active recovery.

A wall-sit is essentially a static negative squat. A 3-second wall-sit is equivalent to doing one body weight squat: 2 seconds down, 1 second up. Thus, a 1-minute wall-sit is 20 squats in 1-minute. Are you up for a 3 or 5 or 7-minute wall-sit challenge? Wall-sits challenge the mind to endure the burn where results literally *begin* to appear. Wall-sits build strength, muscular endurance, and strength of mind. They are among the hardest exercises I have experienced that demand so much fortitude to constantly endure for a length of time. What doesn't kill me, makes me stronger, right? Stay the course and focus!

I can teach a 30-minute wall-sit class consisting of 6 sets of 3-minutes each for 18 minutes. The other 12-minutes consist of 2-minute active recovery periods between each 3-minute wall-sit. I have observed a lot of people doing wall-sits with their feet out in front too far past their knees, and not rather under their knees to actually get into a squat position to feel and stimulate the quads. Granted, modifications are necessary but not at the expense of not feeling the quad muscles of a wall-sit.

People who put their feet out in front past their knees gives them the "illusion" that they did a 3 or 4 or even a 5-minute wall-sit when in fact they did not due to failing to get into a squat position to actually feel the constant burning sensation of the muscle fibers running up and down the quads.

Even when a person is wall-sitting near parallel, if the feet are out too far in front, it can cause the wall-sitter to use the floor with their feet to press their back against the wall to keep "wall-sitting." Be honest with yourself and practice good form with modifications that makes the exercise both safe and effective for you.

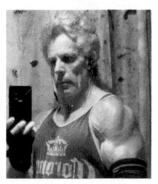 When lockdown was lifted after 51 days, I became a believer in resistance tube training. I became stronger, more muscular and got more defined. Tube training delivers a crazy and unbelievable constant "time under tension," especially at the completion of the concentric part of the movement that challenges the mind to sustain! Tube training is so safe and effective that it is difficult to cheat and injure yourself.

Then the State of Washington declared a second lockdown in fall. For me that meant no haircut again. This was my way of protesting the mandate by letting my hair grow until the gyms reopened like the first lockdown. The day before the gyms were mandated to shut down, I had a 3-hour workout consisting of two workout days into one day because I knew I would miss my iron brothers and sisters.

The gym has been my home away from home for over 40 years. It is an active and energizing environment. It is a place where we can all motivate each other because we all share a common goal: to get stronger, leaner and fitter.

Like everyone else, I had a difficult time because of the mandated COVID-19 restriction a second time around. I had to change my mindset to re-adapt myself to my home environment and get out my resistance tubes to keep exercising.

Advanced Training Techniques

I've always preferred to train alone because I'm always moving. I like to stay focused on stimulating muscle growth and increasing cardiorespiratory endurance. A training partner tends to slow me down. I don't rest until I am finished with my workout. I am focused to train hard to get the job done quickly and efficiently.

The training techniques below can be used when you are training alone. They are: pre-exhaust, supersets, dropsets, burnsets, two-part reps, rest/pause, partial reps, static reps and controlled failure. The last four or five on the list follows a sequential order and can be used for an entire set of an exercise.

Pre-exhaust. This technique pre-exhausts a muscle when performing an "isolation" single-joint movement first before performing a "compound" multiple-joint movement. This is a great technique to use to get past plateaus. It can make "weak points" stronger, which can enable you to use more weight in the bench, squat or deadlift when performed first.

Here are some examples. When training quads start with leg extensions first followed by squats. When training chest start with dumbbell flys first followed by bench press. When training lower back start with back extensions first followed by deadlifts. And when training biceps start with concentration curls first followed by barbell curls.

The point is that pre-exhausting muscles using an isolation exercise first forces the muscles to work harder in a compound exercise because it minimizes secondary muscle involvement (like the shoulders and triceps in bench press and hips in squats and deadlifts) to maximize muscle growth. Pre-exhaust is an excellent technique to break through strength plateaus in compound movements like bench, squats or deadlifts.

Supersets. This is training opposing pushing or "extension" and pulling or "flexion" muscle groups together as one set without rest. After a set of a "push" exercise is complete move on to do a set of a "pull" exercise or vice versa without rest and repeat. Here are some examples: Standing barbell curls → Tricep pushdowns; Leg extensions → Hamstring curls; Bench press → Bent-over barbell rows; and so on.

Burnsets. This is my favorite. It is supersetting the same "push" or "pull" muscle group with a different exercise and movement without rest. It can keep your training localized in one spot or a station until you are done. Burnsets build up a tremendous amount of muscular endurance by burning or fatiguing the muscles quick. You can perform burnsets like you perform supersets or trisets combining two or three exercises together as one set. Here are some examples: Bench press → Dumbbell flys; Bent-over barbell rows → Lat pulldowns; Shoulder press → Side raise; Squats → Leg press; and so on.

Two-Part Reps. This is the same as three-part reps (or 24s) except the movement for the exercise is done in two parts rather than three. The movement begins at the weakest range of motion (ROM) and ends with the strongest ROM. The entire execution transitions from weakest ROM to strongest ROM. Let look at two exercises: seated barbell curls to standing barbell curls and seated barbell front raises to standing barbell front raises.

Curl the weight in a seated position from mid-point to full flexion. After completing a predetermined number of reps immediately stand up and curl the weight from bottom to mid-point. For front raises, raise the weight from mid-point to full extension. After completing a predetermined number of reps immediately stand up and raise the weight from bottom to mid-point. The same can be performed doing side raises.

Dropsets or Descending Sets. This is a popular technique. It is like reverse pyramid training but performed as one set. Do as many reps as you can do with a weight. Without rest grab a lighter weight or decrease the weight and do the same, and so on until you can't perform any more reps in good form. That's one set. You can use this technique by training to failure using the subsequent techniques below to continue.

Rest/Pause. This is like a self-help forced rep. Say you want to squeeze out a few more reps of an exercise, but you can't because your muscles are naturally fatigued by your super awesome form. Sit-up, put the weight down or rack the weight. Rest for 10 to 15 seconds. Catch your breath and psych yourself up before continuing where you left off to finish the set with 2 to 3 more reps than if you didn't rest/pause.

Partial Reps. You are not quite finished with your set after you do your rest/pause reps. You have more in you because your muscles are physically screaming for more! So, what do you do if you cannot do a full rep? Do partial reps. Partial reps are performed when you can no longer do full reps but can still move the weight. First, three-quarter reps. Then, half reps. Next, one-third reps. After that, one-quarter reps. And finally, when you can no longer *move* the weight.

Static Reps. But wait! Just because you can't move the weight you can still physically hold the weight for a few seconds more in a position of muscular contraction and statically dig deep into every ounce of muscle fiber to full mental and physical exhaustion.

Controlled Failure. Congratulations! You've reached controlled failure! That last set was grueling. You went from doing full reps, to dropsets, to rest/pause, to partial reps, to static reps, and finally to controlled failure in superb form! The limbs of your body cannot move because you've forced the muscles to adapt to the stress. They only have one option: to get stronger and bigger.

Seeking Failure

Will Smith says that people usually have a negative relationship with failure. But failure, he says, is a huge part of being able to be successful. You must get comfortable with failure. You must actually seek failure. Failure is where all of the lessons are learned. He wittingly says that when you go to the gym and workout you are actually seeking failure. You want to take your muscles to a "controlled failure" because failure is where the adaptation is, where growth is.

Successful people fail a lot, but they extract the lessons from failure and they use the energy and the wisdom to come around to the next phase of success. You have to live where for almost certain you are going to fail. Failure helps you recognize the areas where you need to evolve. Fail early, fail often, fail forward.[77]

Training Precautions when Exercising Alone

One day at the gym in the late 90s an older fellow said to me, "You sure are quiet when you have a catastrophe!"

I was benching 245 pounds with the collars on, but on the fifth rep I got stuck at mid-point and the weight slowly descended. This older fellow was supposed to be spotting me, but he happened to be looking the other direction talking to his buddy. But before the bar made contact with my chest, I slowly lowered the 245-pound loaded bar down to my mid-section. Within a half a second, I used the weight to pull myself up and sit up. Within another half second, I rolled the bar down onto my thighs and stood up grasping the heavy weighted bar before resting it on the end of the bench. This is what you can do if you are alone doing bench press with collars on to *save your life!*

If you fail doing squats and not using a squat rack, you can do one of two things to save your knees or your life. One, keep the collars off. Keeping the collars off will enable you to tilt the bar to one side and slide the weight off and then the other side (also for bench press). Two, do what the athletes do with Olympic lifts: let go of the bar and quickly move forward to have gravity do its thing and let the weight drop to the floor behind you.

Muscle Soreness

Almost everyone who has ever lifted weights has experienced some type of muscle soreness. Generally, muscle soreness associated with weight training can be broken down into two categories: acute muscle soreness (AMS) and delayed-onset muscle soreness (DOMS).

AMS is that "burning" sensation that you feel during exercise from a buildup of lactic acid in the muscle. AMS is thought to be associated with a lack of adequate blood flow to the active muscles. Because of the diminished blood flow to the working muscles, waste products such as lactic acid and potassium cannot be removed from the muscle and begin to accrue within the muscle. It is this build-up of metabolic waste products that is thought to stimulate pain receptors located within the muscles.

The "burn" does not necessarily mean that the muscles are being worked any harder, only that blood flow to the muscle is being reduced. The acute burning pain continues until the intensity of the contraction is reduced or stopped and blood flow is restored allowing removal of the accumulated waste products. Regularly exercised muscles better tolerate and dispose the accumulated waste products.

DOMS is caused by damage to the muscle fibers. DOMS appears the day after exercise and gets worse after the second day before dissipating. When muscle is damaged from a training session it is important to consume protein. Protein re-builds the damaged muscles by making them thicker, stronger, and bigger.

It is interesting to point out that *lack of soreness* is not an indication that you didn't have a positive training experience and that you are not producing favorable environmental factors to stimulate muscle growth. The "feeling" of soreness is a result of pain receptors being triggered due to inflammation and since people have different responses to pain, we cannot use this as a measure for a "good" workout.

I once knew someone that when he trained his chest never felt sore the next day yet made muscular gains. Why? He did two important things outside the gym. He followed a high-performance nutrition plan and always got a sufficient amount of recuperation.

It is very easy to over-train a small body part like the biceps. The name of the muscle game is to stimulate, not annihilate. Because most young guys want big biceps, they fall into the trap thinking more is better. When training biceps take 8x Mr. Olympia Lee Haney's advice, "Feel them, pump them, and move on."

The "No Pain, No Gain" dictum can be self-defeating. There is such a thing as over-working your muscles. You can actually traumatize and damage the muscle fibers to such an extent that they have been over-worked and not be able to recuperate for weeks.

Does Hypertrophy Stop at Age 40?

Muscle does not know age. It is true that when a person ages, hormone production lessens, which makes muscular gains slower and more difficult. However, it is well known that additional muscle can be acquired by a beginner exerciser at almost any age. If the person has been training for many years and has already added a significant amount of muscle, progress is usually slower than in the case of the beginner. When one ages, one needs more time to recuperate after an intense workout. One also needs to be more diligent with diet since metabolism naturally slows down with age. But with age comes wisdom. Hard work, dedication and sound nutritional information are the foundation of a complete fitness package. Putting your goals in proper perspective assists in guiding you toward furthering your pursuit of fitness.

Most people never reach their fitness goals because of incorrect eating and training and insufficient recuperation. If you are lifting with proper form, stimulating enough exercise stress, eating properly and getting sufficient rest, then you will get results. There is no basis to support the myth that muscle hypertrophy ends at a certain age.

Training Journal

Some people carry their phones around in the gym performing a routine prescribed by someone they are following on social media or carry their prescribed training program with them and record the same thing they did day in and day out: exercise, weight, sets, reps.

What I do is that I carry a piece of paper with a "game plan" already drafted telling me what I should do that workout to keep making progress. Before I leave for the gym, I open my training journal and review my previous workout. On a blank piece of paper, I write down what goals I should strive for in this workout.

When I get back home after the workout, I record what I actually did. A training journal is pro-active and is made up of two parts: (1) a drafted game plan and (2) a record of what was actually done in that workout. Never come to the gym empty handed not knowing what you are going to do.

A training journal is a tool. It provides a chart of your progress when you are training and keeps you on top of your game. It can include how you felt before, during and after your workout. It allows you to see your strength increases, weaknesses, injuries.

A training journal keeps you motivated. It keeps you alert. It keeps you positive. It helps you to train smart. It keeps you stay focused and committed. It tells you when to adjust your weight, change exercises, sets, reps, what to do, what not to do, how to do it, etc.

A training journal helps you to plan each and every workout so you will be able to see the *process of your desired goal in each workout.*

Enjoyment, Low-Impact, Good Form

A quick-paced high-impact workout with less attention on form and where joint alignment cannot be monitored is a cause for reflection in regard to safety.

I took a Boot Camp class early in the morning for a week and a half for five 30-minute sessions. Even though it kicked my butt and I saw noticeable results in such a short time I stopped doing it because I got burned out. It was neither fun nor safe. In my opinion, there are three things that high-impact intense exercise modalities fail to satisfy for most people: enjoyment, low-impact, and good form.

It is true that moving quickly between exercises is important to keep the training intense for effecting the calorie and fat burn during and after exercise, but not at the expense of improper form with too much weight (even one's body weight alone) over time from doing high-impact modality exercises (e.g., box jumps, burpees, kettlebell swings, etc.).

Some exercise enthusiasts quit these types of classes and sabotage their fitness because they can no longer exercise due to developing knee injuries, shoulder injuries, back injuries, wrist injuries, elbow injuries, ankle injuries, and even plantar fasciitis.

Injuries

Injuries, whether prolonged, sustained or immediate, can be caused by a number of factors regardless of training routine. Look out for these: (1) insufficient warm-up, (2) poor exercise form, (3) lack of full-range movements, (4) joint or tendon overuse with or without the presence of pain, (5) improperly positioned joints, (6) increasing weight too quickly, (7) lack of rest, (8) utilizing advanced weight training techniques too often, (9) not cycling training intensity, (10) poor focus or lack of concentration, (11) lack of proper nutrition, (12) overstraining a muscle with too much weight, (13) hyperextending a joint or tendon, (14) ignoring localized pain. The list is inexhaustive. Injuries to joints and tendons are usually more prevalent than muscles.

A common injury among bodybuilders, weightlifters and powerlifters is Carpal Tunnel Syndrome (CTS). It is a painful condition caused by the median nerve on the palm side of the wrist being repeatedly and frequently compressed.

Because weightlifters use their hands and wrists extensively, they often exhibit traditional CTS symptoms. To prevent CTS, you can do three things: (1) avoid jerking your wrists while lifting, (2) schedule your workouts so you don't overwork your hands or wrists, and (3) use wrist wraps for extra support. If this fails and you start developing symptoms of CTS see a doctor.

Injury Prevention

Stretch! Stretching should optimally be done during and after training, not before. There are two types of basic stretching movements: dynamic and static.

Dynamic stretching is the type used in sports and activities like soccer, cycling, tennis, basketball, rock climbing, etc. It is performed before starting the actual sport or activity. It consists of the exerciser "actively" stretching the muscles through repeated short-range movements to increase strength, flexibility and performance.

Static stretching is the type used in weight training. It is or should be performed after completing a training session. It consists of the exerciser "passively" holding the stretched position for 30-60 seconds and repeating two more times.

Performing static stretches prior to exercise *can* reduce muscle tension and its ability to fire and contract because the muscle fibers are relaxed. This relaxed tension can alter the length-tension relationship of the muscle and cause a decrease in muscle excitability. This can affect the muscle's ability to optimally function and can decrease overall performance during exercise. Stretching before exercise *may* either cause an injury to the muscle or sabotage a training session altogether.

In weight training, you can stretch either after completing a muscle group or training session. You may stretch between sets of an exercise or exercises of the same muscle group but then again, this might prematurely cause the muscle to relax and decrease performance for the remaining sets.

It is best to stretch after completing a muscle group before moving on to the next one. Stretching after completing a muscle group or training session can help relieve cramping and *initiate* the recuperation process and prevent injuries.

Exercising the quadricep muscles every day by following a full body weight training and cardio routine can cause them to tighten and cramp up frequently at night. It's a scary incident and it's painful.

Magnesium is used for many things, but I discovered that taking a 500mg capsule after a workout helps to relax the nerves in the leg muscles to prevent cramping. Taking liquid magnesium may help to relieve cramps immediately.

Training Through an Injury

In most cases, but not all, it is better to train through an injury, granted that it is not serious or severe that it needs medical attention. It is important to approach injuries on their own terms. First, pinpoint the injury. Second, know why you got the injury. And third, modify your training (lighter weight, different exercise, better warm-up) to help heal the injury.

Be smart and protect injuries when training or prevent new ones from occurring in order to still make improvements to your body. Wear a lifting belt and put on knee wraps when squatting heavy. Wear elbow sleeves when benching or pressing. Wear wrist wraps when weight lifting. Use lifting straps, hooks or liquid chalk for reinforcing your grip.

Training through an injury can cause three beneficial things: (1) helps the injury and surrounding tissue maintain strength, (2) prevents the injury and surrounding tissue from becoming cold and atrophying, and (3) keeps the injury strong so it does not become susceptible to further injury.

One word of advice: When you begin to feel sharp acute pain in the elbows, knees, shoulders or wrists and if you are stubborn enough to train through them even harder and they get worse, STOP! Re-evaluate your training to keep your ego in check to avoid further injuries or prolonging old injuries to heal. Train smart.

R.I.C.E Method

Injuries associated with joint pain, minor muscle pulls, severe muscle strains or tendon discomfort use the R.I.C.E. method to keep the swelling down and under control to speed up the healing.

R.I.C.E stands for Rest, Ice, Compression, Elevation. Rest is the obvious start of the healing process. Elevate the injured part, apply Ice and Compress it. Elevating the injured area preferably above the heart ensures blood circulation to and from the heart.

Apply the 15-on and 45-off system. That is, ice the injured part for 15 minutes, followed by 45 minutes without ice. The ice might start to sting a bit only after applying it for a few minutes. This might be because the injury is deep and severe. That's okay. If the ice starts to "burn" the injured area too much, then remove it for a minute or two before re-applying it.

You must become your own sports medicine doctor by listening to your own body to know how to treat common injuries. Omit some exercises, incorporate new exercises and change your routine, but keep exercising. If you are in doubt what to do or your injuries worsen seek medical advice!

Body Types and Training Plans

Before you decide how you will train by selecting which exercises are best for you to do, it is important that you take a look at yourself and categorize yourself into one of three body types: (1) ectomorph, (2) endomorph or (3) mesomorph. A person may be a combination of two types, e.g., an ecto-mesomorph.

An ectomorph is a thin person with light bone structure and long tenuous muscles. The ectomorph has a hard time building strength and gaining muscle. An ectomorph is an ideal runner. An endomorph is a stocky person with thick bones and tends to be round and stout. The endomorph can gain weight fast and be able to handle heavy training but difficult to get definition. An endomorph is an ideal powerlifter. A mesomorph is an athletic-looking person who has a large frame, the capacity for becoming muscular fast and the ability to get defined. A mesomorph is an ideal bodybuilder.

Everyone can improve his or her body regardless of body type. If you are an ectomorph, then you probably have a fast metabolism. And you need to eat more food at regular times to gain weight. If you are an endomorph you may have to monitor what, how much and how often you eat to avoid fat gain. If you are a mesomorph, the athletic, muscular type, you might achieve outstanding physical performance and a great physique.

Unless the ectomorph is training as a long-distance runner for endurance, the type of training plan for an ectomorph wanting to gain weight would consist of performing basic compound movements with heavy weight and moderate reps, resting longer between sets and training days and eating high-calorie foods frequently.

Unless the endomorph is training as a powerlifter to gain weight for strength and power, the type of training plan for an endomorph wanting to lose weight would consist of performing basic compound movements with moderate weight and high reps, supersetting between exercises, training more often during the week and eating low-calorie foods frequently.

The type of training plan for a mesomorph would consist of adopting both types of training plans of the ectomorph to gain weight and endomorph to gain strength and power and to lose weight, but at different times during the year conducive to the desired goal.

Full-Body vs. Split Routines

Three basic *progressive training routines* are considered that should be followed based on experience, fitness goal and the best buck for time and consistency. First, the 3-day full-body routine whereby one trains the whole body three times a week. Second, the 4-day split routine whereby one trains half the body one day and the other half the body the next day. Each muscle group is trained two times a week. And third, the 5 to 6-day split routine whereby one trains one or two muscle groups in a workout. Each muscle group is trained approximately once a week.

Generally speaking, each routine is a graduation from one routine to the other in terms of experience and training intensity. But it also depends on how many days a week one is committed to training in light of a specific goal and purpose of the routine.

The 3-day full-body routine typically follows a Monday, Wednesday, Friday plan. The 4-day split routine typically follows a Monday/Thursday and Tuesday/Friday plan whereby you train the same muscle groups on the days designated by the slash between them. The 5 to 6-day split routine has variable training days in regard to how the exerciser plans it for the week. One can either train a muscle group or muscle groups on a fixed day during the week or choose a training plan with no fixed days by adopting a 2-ON, 1-OFF or a 3-ON, 1 or 2-OFF weekly schedule. The exerciser would either train two straight days and take one day off and repeat or train three straight days and take one day or two days off and repeat.

If you are limited with time and want to improve your whole physique equally and improve your fitness, then the 3-day a week full-body weight routine can provide the most value for your time and effort.

There are three main advantages of full-body routines. One, if you have limited time during the week, then the whole body is trained. Two, multi-joint or compound exercises compared to isolation or single-joint exercises are more effective in full-body routines because more work is performed in less time and more energy is expended (more calories are burned).

And three, missing a workout does not necessarily set you back because you've already trained all of your muscle groups twice that week. Now if you miss a workout on a split routine, it means that you neglected a particular muscle group that week and it would be nearly two weeks until it is trained again.

Full-body routines work. They are holistic routines. If you also incorporate a full-body cardio routine during the week, then both routines allow you to train every day, which can condition and improve the body daily and rest days become optional. A full-body weight training routine allows each muscle group to be trained frequently and equally during the week. So, you can be rest assured that if you miss a workout, you will still be ahead of the game to bettering your fitness.

If you want to maximize your time, your effort, your calories and want to see weekly improvements in strength, core stabilization, functional mobility, endurance, and a higher caloric burn, then full-body routines get the upper hand.

General Training Variables

Experience of "consistency"	Beginner (0-6 months)	Intermediate (6-18 months)	Advanced (1 ½ + years)
Routine type	3-day a week full-body	4-day a week split-body	5-6 day a week split-body
Muscle groups trained per week	3 times	2 times	1-2 times
Sets per workout	4 (large) 3 (small)	6 (large) 5 (small)	6-12 (large) 5-10 (small)
Rests (between sets)	90 seconds to 2 minutes	60-90 seconds	30-60 seconds
Rests (between days)	1-2 days	2-3 days	2-6 days

Not What Kind, But *How* You Exercise

People are mistaken saying that weight training does not give a calorie burn like high-impact exercise modalities. The mistake rests on the image *how* weight training is conventionally performed these days, which is "anaerobically," i.e., without the presence of oxygen.

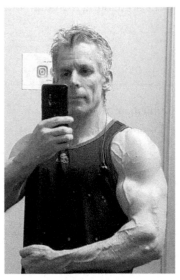

But if your primary goal is to lose fat *and* build muscle quicker, then you must train for *muscular and cardiorespiratory endurance* and train practically every day at a steady-state of 80-90% for at least 45 minutes. This kind of training can give you a calorie and after-burn like no other!

Time *and* intensity go hand-in-hand to build muscle *and* lose fat simultaneously – coupled with post-exercise nutrition and sufficient recuperation. You can measure your weight training intensity by dividing the total number of repetitions you do in a training session into the time it takes to complete a training session. For example, say you did 35 sets and 600 repetitions in 60 minutes. This turns out to be 10 repetitions every minute! You must be willing to put in your work to be the cause of the changes. After all, "If it doesn't challenge you, it doesn't change you."[78]

Some people might ask, "Well, don't you need a day or two of rest to recover?" My answer is no, not necessarily. Working out 60 minutes 7 days a week *only* makes up 4% of the entire week. The other 96% accounts for the recovery process; "rest periods" if you will. When this is broken down to 60-minute workouts a day ask yourself, "What am I doing in the 23 hours after exercise to recover?" The first phase of recovery occurs 30-90 minutes after exercise. The second phase of recovery occurs 2-4 hours after exercise. And the third phase of recovery occurs 48-72 hours after exercise.

I have been frequently approached by people who ask me which cardio machine is better to burn more calories. First, people shouldn't be looking for a certain machine to burn a lot of calories because a machine doesn't to do it for you. How many calories you want to burn is up to how much energy you put out while exercising.

Second, people must focus on creating a longer after-burn when they are exercising so that their bodies *can* burn more calories after exercise, even at rest. A higher calorie after-burn after exercise can only be accomplished by a steady-state range with an intensity high enough to keep the body's metabolism elevated days after a training session. A shorter duration means a higher intensity since more work is accomplished in less time for a longer after-burn.

And third, for those who ask me which cardio machine burns the most calories my response is always the same, "It's not what you do that burns calories, but *how* you do it." Don't leave it up to a certain machine to burn calories. It is up to you *how* you use it.

Self-Discipline is Freedom

One of my pet peeves is people confusing work with exercise as an excuse NOT to exercise. First, exercise elevates the heart rate. Second, the body starts to overheat. And third, sweat and toxins from inside the body will start dissipating from the skin trying to cool and cleanse itself. Exercise is hard work. But like a lot of things if you want to get somewhere and succeed, it requires self-discipline. After all, "No pain, no change."

Will Smith talks about self-discipline as self-love. When you say you love yourself that means you have behavior towards yourself that is loving. You say to yourself I know you want to eat that pizza and you know it will taste good, but I can't let you do that because I love you too much. It is not discipline in the sense of punishment, but discipline in the sense that you forgo immediate pleasure for the exchange of long-term self-respect.

At the center for bringing any dream into fruition is self-discipline. It is getting command of your mind for choosing actions in your own best interest. You cannot win the war against the world if you cannot win the war against your own mind.[79] Choosing to exercise is in your best interest! Choosing a safe exercise modality is in your best interest! Choosing to stay committed is in your best interest! Command your mind and your body will follow. Exercise repeatedly and you will know how to *exercise well*.

What Does it Mean to Exercise Well?

Even if we know how to exercise, we cannot exercise well if we do not know how each muscle functions in relation to the direction of how it moves each limb on the body and apply it to each exercise.[80]

Exercising to exercising better to exercising well is a process. It requires repeated acts of the same exercise movement to make it more precise and efficient for physiological changes to occur. This is why exercising is 80% and nutrition 20%. The benefits from exercise alone are noted above.[81]

Signs that you are exercising better to exercising well to effect changes to the body in regard to why we exercise[82] include: (1) you feel better than when you started, (2) the exercises feel easier to do, (3) you are more coordinated, (4) you are able to have better form, (5) you are able to move through a greater range of motion, (6) you are able to challenge yourself by making the exercise harder rather than going through the motions, (7) you are feeling your muscles working more, (8) you are able to train longer or more intense, (9) you have a feeling of accomplishment after, and (10) you are looking forward to the next workout session.[83]

Fun, Safe and Long-Term

What shall we say about weight resistance training? Can it give you a calorie burn like CrossFit, Boot Camps and TRX? The answer is a resounding yes! Weight training is low-impact because *you are in control of your environment.* High-intensity training is how well you are able to perform each rep of each set of the exercise to stimulate an X number of fibers at that time. Weight resistance training requires a full range of motion in a controlled manner while maintaining good form. It is up to you how you weight train for the results you want.

Habit #5

Adopt a Useful Exercise Modality for the Rest of Your Life

CHAPTER 6

REVERSE PYRAMID TRAINING

Become limitless *by adopting the train hard, not long mentality for quicker results.*

People generally use one of these three weight training methods for increasing strength, gaining muscle, and losing fat: (1) ascending pyramid training, (2) five by five training or (3) reverse pyramid training. These are called "methods" because each is a process by which some end is achieved.

Ascending Pyramid Training

This is by far the most popular training method and has been for nearly a century. Ascending pyramid training is the method whereby you pyramid up in weight (increase the weight) with each successive set while your reps decrease because of muscle fatigue. It is a great method for the beginner or anyone at any level of training. I used ascending pyramid training when I first started lifting weights at home to gain weight while in my teens.

Let's use the bench press for an example in how this method is used. Some do five sets, but let's do three sets. Do your first set with

135 pounds for 15 reps. Do your second set with 155 pounds for 12 reps. And do your third and final set with 185 pounds for 8 reps.

A person might do one or two more sets for maybe 6, then 4 reps. Normally, you would stop there, and you should before you move to your next exercise.

But some people, after pyramiding up in weight and pyramiding down in reps, like to continue training in reverse (reverse pyramid) until they are at their original weight (or lower) than they started.

For example, they might do a fourth (or sixth) set with 155 pounds for as many reps they can do. And then, a fifth (or seventh) set with 135 pounds for as many reps as they can do. And possibly, one more, a sixth (or eighth) set, with 115 pounds for as many reps as they can do in order to "burn out."

Overtraining

But the "more is better" dictum at any experienced level of training may prove to be self-defeating. If post-exercise stress is excessive on the body, and it is *not* met with post-exercise nutrition and sufficient recovery, then the body will not be able to supercompensate.

Strength and muscle gains will begin to decrease or come to a screeching halt. This is what happens when the body enters an over-trained state. See the diagram on the following page. The corresponding numbers match the numbers in the diagram.

But anyone using any training method can be susceptible to overtraining. Keep in mind that an extra day or two of rest is more beneficial to the body than an extra day or two of training sessions. When tired one day or in doubt take a day off. Listen to your body.

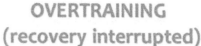

OVERTRAINING
(recovery interrupted)

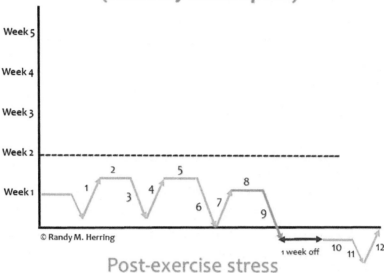

Week 5

Week 4

Week 3

Week 2

Week 1

© Randy M. Herring

1 week off

Post-exercise stress

Restoration toward supercompensation (as indicated by the -------) from the previous workout is pre-maturely interrupted (1). Workout volume is mistakenly increased; muscular strength occurs but is leveling off at week two (2). Because of insufficient recovery time stress gradually and dangerously builds up (3). The body positively reacts to the additional stress by compensating for it due to permitted rest but cannot yet supercompensate (-------) (4). Strength and muscle gains level off and a plateau is realized at week three (5). A lack of sufficient rest for two weeks is causing undo stress on the body, and, as a result, it weakens and becomes prone to injury (6).

The body's recuperative ability negates post-exercise stress due to a lack of rest (7). After week four, strength and muscle gains decrease and an overtraining state is realized (8). Post-exercise stress becomes increasingly potent and impossible for any length of recovery to benefit until you are forced to *take a week off* at week five so the body can catch up with itself to recover from the over-trained state (9). Training resumes at week six (10).

Post-exercise stress occurs and damage to tissues naturally follows (11). Post-exercise rest and high-performance nutrition aids in healing the damaged muscle fibers so they can become stronger. The body recovers and inherently "bounces-back." Restoration toward supercompensation can once again be realized heading into week seven (12).

Five by Five Training

Five by five training or 5x5 is used by bodybuilders and athletes to build strength and muscle. This type of training is designed for those who have a solid foundation in the basic compound exercises and whose intensity is much higher than the beginner.

A person performs five compound exercises each week three times a week: deadlift, squat, bench press, overhead press, and barbell row. It consists of two different workouts (A & B) that are rotated during the week on Monday (Day 1), Wednesday (Day 2), and Friday (Day 3).

Monday (Day1) includes Barbell Squats, Barbell Bench Press, and Bent-over Barbell Rows. Wednesday (Day 2) includes Front Barbell Squats, Standing Military Press, and Barbell Deadlift. Friday (Day 3) includes Barbell Squats, Barbell Bench Press, and Bent-over Barbell Rows. Workout A is performed on Days 1 and 3. And workout B is performed on Day 2.

Find your proper weight that you are able to perform for a total of 25 reps per exercise. Gradually increase your weight to maximize strength and muscle gains. For example, it is recommended to increase the weight by five pounds on dumbbells and by ten pounds on each side on barbell exercises.

Since this system is a method of maximum weight overload on the body it can be taxing on the whole body, even the nervous system. For this reason, the biggest disadvantage with type of training is that you may experience prolonged recovery times and, potentially, the risk of overtraining, as described in the diagram above.

Reverse Pyramid Training (RPT)

The popular ascending pyramid training method is neither energy nor time efficient. Pyramiding up in weight while pyramiding down in reps wastes time, energy, and muscular effort. A pragmatic training approach that is energy and time efficient is the reverse pyramid. Reverse pyramid training turns the ascending pyramid method upside down and reverses the weight and rep scheme.

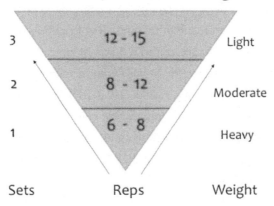

Reverse Pyramid Training

Sets	Reps	Weight
3	12 - 15	Light
2	8 - 12	Moderate
1	6 - 8	Heavy

Rather than beginning with the lightest weight and doing 12 repetitions for the first set you'll reverse the order and begin your first set with the heaviest weight you can handle for 8 repetitions since this is when you are fresh and strongest. For each succeeding set you will decrease the weight (pyramid down in weight, hence, the "reverse" pyramid) and increase the reps.

Why RPT?

I am unsure how "reverse pyramid training" got its name, but it seems to stem from Arthur Jones' application of high-intensity training with the late Mr. Universe Mike Mentzer in the 70s. So, it appears reasonable to say that it has been around for over 50 years.

Mentzer adapted Jones' HIT to his training system and called it "Heavy-Duty." According to Mentzer, building muscle is directly related to intensity, not duration (against high-volume training). He based his idea on biology and physiology.

Six-time Mr. Olympia, Dorian Yates, became a proponent of Mentzer's heavy-duty system in the 90s. He adapted it to one all out "high-intensity" set to failure and called it "Blood and Guts."

I never did follow Mentzer or Yates, but the *train hard, not long* idea made more sense to me than training long. I put this idea into practice in the latter 90s and adapted it to 2-3 sets of an exercise, rather than 4-5 sets, which is characteristic of high-volume training.

After six months, my results using RPT as a "hardgainer" and ectomorph blew me away. I built muscle quicker in a shorter amount of time than using the ascending pyramid training method. Bench press increased by 35% for a 300-pound 1RM. Incline bench press increased by 30% for a 185-pound 10RM. Weighted dips increased by 35% with 3 plates attached to my waist. Seated press behind the neck increased for a 135-pound 10RM. And my biceps girth increased by one-fourth of an inch in less than a month.

I was confident that this training approach could be implemented by anyone wanting to build muscle quicker! Three years later, near the turn of the millennium, I had written an unpublished spiral bound 240-page book called *Reverse Pyramid Training: And The Fifteen Rules For*

Building Lean Muscle Mass. I shared this proven and sensible training method on the World Wide Web to help other "hardgainers" like myself to make quicker gains. Book sales were quite successful.

Train Hard, Not Long

Building muscle encompasses three basic facts. One, strength precedes muscle. Before a muscle can get bigger it first must get stronger.

Two, training hard and long is impossible. You either train hard or long. You cannot do both. Training harder means training at a higher intensity and invariably shortens your workout time. It doesn't necessarily mean using heavier weight, but rather making a set harder to complete, which brings us to the third fact.

And three, the greater amount of force generated yields the most muscle fibers stimulated at one time. This is the "time under tension" principle. The amount of force you make a muscle generate is directly proportional to the potential amount of muscle growth.

RPT Benefits

RPT offers a number of incomparable benefits for those who want to stop wasting countless hours, energy, and muscular effort in the gym. One, fewer sets are proposed than the conventional ascending pyramid. Two, training time is decreased by half because of a greater amount of intensity. Three, training hard, not long renders a more efficient and productive training session. Four, greater recuperative ability is afforded to your muscles, thus, permitting them to get stronger and bigger quicker. And five, more attention to concentration and effort is demanded, which forces the mind to grow and get stronger with each subsequent body transformation.

Physiology and Psychology of the Reverse

Since the first set will be your heaviest weight the physiology of the reverse is that your energy will be freshest and you will be stronger than if you used the same weight for the last set using the ascending pyramid. If a set counts it's this one!

The psychology is that it is easier going down than up. The weight not only will seem lighter on your last set but it will be lighter. It is refreshing to know that the last set is your last chance to use all your muscles to train to fatigue in order to stimulate muscle growth after the workout.

Each descending set is like a warm-down but just as intense. That is to say, you will experience strength increases on your third and last set just as you will on your first and second sets. So, warm-downs help monitor strength increases, whereby you can end up with a heavier warm-down set than when you first started.

Modifying the Reverse Pyramid

The 6, 8, 10 reverse pyramid rep system is good for increasing strength and building muscle. But as you can see in the Reverse Pyramid Training diagram above the rep scheme can be modified to suit your fitness needs and sport specific goals.

Suppose you want to build muscle *and* lose fat. Simply change your rep scheme to 10, 12, 15. Superset between exercises and rest no more than 30 seconds between each superset. For specific strength training for a sport like football change your rep scheme to 4, 6, 8, and rest 2-5 minutes between sets. Practically anybody can benefit from reverse pyramid training. It all depends on how reverse pyramid training is utilized for a desired goal.

Genetics: High-Volume vs High-Intensity

Every person who trains intelligently can make improvements. As mentioned above, each person's body type is either classified as an ectomorph, endomorph or mesomorph. Each person is also predisposed to having a certain percentage of predominant *slow-twitch* muscle fibers (type I) or *fast-twitch* muscle fibers (type II) designated for endurance or power, respectively. So, genetics does play a role in what kind of *training system* works best for you to build muscle.

Most bodybuilders have been successful building muscle using high-volume training like Arnold Schwarzenegger whereas few bodybuilders have been successful building muscle using high-intensity training (HIT), specifically, Dorian Yates. These are called training "systems" because they are based on principles that incorporate a method of training. The former is a part of a whole, so to speak.

Arnold popularized high-volume training in the 70s. It can be characterized in terms of the *quantity* of "the pump" and described as a moderate training system. Unverified by Arnold himself, Internet sources claim he trained for one hour a day, six days a week and trained each muscle group two times per week. He performed supersets of three to four sets of each exercise for at least 10 reps before reaching failure. He did anywhere from 25-60 sets in a workout for large muscle groups. Arnold is classified as a mesomorph and most likely has a predominance of slow-twitch muscle fibers (type I) for endurance training. This is why high-volume training worked best for him.[84]

High-volume training is more popular because it is more enjoyable, recovery is faster, and less apt to get injured. Arnold is considered for having the best physique of all time based on size, symmetry, small waist, definition and aesthetics. He was 6 foot, 2 inches and weighed 235 pounds at competition.

Dorian, who credits the late Mike Mentzer's "Heavy-Duty" principles to his training, took Arthur Jones' high-intensity training to a whole new level in the 90s. It can be characterized in terms of the *quality* of "maximum muscle stimulation" and described as an extreme training system.

Unverified by Dorian himself, Internet sources claim he trained one hour a day, four days a week and trained each muscle group once a week. He performed one all out working set of an exercise for at least 6 reps before continuing to train to failure using partial reps, forced reps and negative reps. Dorian is classified as an endo-mesomorph and most likely has a predominance of fast-twitch muscle fibers (type II) for explosive-power training. This is why HIT worked best for him.

High-intensity training "Dorian style" seems less popular because it is brutally intense, recovery is slower, and more apt to get injured. Dorian is considered the first "mass monster" in bodybuilding. He had hard dense muscle and was shredded at contest shape. He was 5 foot, 10 inches and weighed 275 pounds at competition.

What does this say about what kind of training system is best for you? First, determine the classification of your body type. Second, subject yourself to both types of training systems. This will take time as you will be adjusting the amount of weight and rep scheme to find out *how much* and *what range* works for you. And third, discover the predominance of your muscle fiber types using the training system that best suits your genetics in regard to point number two.

RPT: High-Volume *and* High-Intensity

One of the beauties of RPT is that it can either be high-volume or high-intensity depending on amount of weight and rep range. I classify myself as an ectomorph with predominately slow-twitch muscle fibers. This gives me the reason *why* my body responds better to high-volume reverse pyramid training.

One or Five vs Three Sets

An article quoted an ESPN Gold's Gym study at the turn of the millennium showed that strength increases on the first (27%) set are more significant than the second (24%) and third (16%) sets.[85] This article seems to support the philosophy behind the 3-set reverse pyramid training scheme by doing the heaviest set first in your workout to generate strength and stimulate muscle gains quicker.

Yet, if one-set proved consistent results for strength increases combined with increased physical fitness more people would be doing it. The reality is, however, that most people want more than strength or desire something other than strength alone: muscle and cardiorespiratory fitness.

Strength gains are prime between 4-6 repetitions. Muscle gains are prime between 8-12 repetitions. Muscular endurance combined with cardiorespiratory conditioning for fat loss are prime between 15-20 repetitions. In my opinion, performing at least two sets assists with both strength and muscle gains.

The disadvantage of performing only one set of an exercise depresses the psychological benefits of exercise: the fun, the heightened vitality, and "the magic of the pump." In addition, incorporating advanced techniques, such as forced reps, negatives and training to failure takes all the fun out of training. It becomes drudgery for those wishing to pursue fitness for a lifetime while remaining injury free.

Strength increases are real to both the ESPN/Gold's Gym study and reverse pyramid training. Executing the first set *and* following two subsequent sets with increasing repetitions demonstrates both significant strength and muscle gains.

However, training "too hard" and too short by doing one-set of an exercise or training "too little" and too long by doing more than 5-sets of an exercise is no fun and can lead to a psychological and self-defeating total burn out.

Performing three sets is a happy Aristotelian medium, not too many in excess like five sets and not too few in deficiency like one set. The goal is to pump up the muscles and exhaust them as quickly and effectively as possible using three sets.

But suppose one day you are having a superb flow experience while exercising. Your endorphins are kicking in, you tax the body to its limit and thoroughly exhaust the muscles in only two sets. Why prolong the exercise, train longer and do another? Making one set count as two sets and one rep count as two reps *is* intensity. Accomplishing more in less time is what high-intensity is all about.

Measuring Intensity with 3-Set RPT

Knowing how much weight you lifted in three sets in a *specific duration of time* can be a practical way to measure "time under tension" and discover how hard you trained (or not). Say you used a moderate weight on your first set of squats for 8 to 12 repetitions, a moderate-light weight on your second set for 15 repetitions, and finally, a light weight on your third set for 20 repetitions.

Suppose you did your first set with 225 pounds for 12 non-stop repetitions. Your next and second set you did 185 pounds for 15 non-stop repetitions. And your last and third set you did 135 pounds for 20 non-stop repetitions. The total time is 8 minutes.

The total number of repetitions is 47. The total amount of weight squatted times repetitions in a full-range of motion is 8,175. The total time to complete 47 repetitions and squat 8,175 pounds in three sets is 8 minutes.

8,175 pounds divided by time duration amounts to nearly 6 repetitions of 1,022 pounds every minute for 8 minutes, which amounts to the duration of "time under tension" for a pumped and fatigued quad workout performing squats and taxing the whole body.

The harder you train in less time means that the muscles fatigue quicker, which can stimulate growth and increase performance faster. The only way to see your progress is if you did this same kind of training again, preferably doing more repetitions with the same weight but in less time.

Conventional Rep Range

The 8-12 rep range is a standard guide for gaining both strength and muscle. But this rep range, like the standard 3 sets of 10 reps, is not written in stone. If you've got more strength and energy to go beyond 8 reps for your first set, then by all means do 2 or 3 more reps! And the same goes for your second and third sets.

Say, for example, you had the strength and energy to do 3 more reps than your usual 12 reps on your third and final set. This means that you've gained an increase in strength and muscle on your "warm-down" set. This is an example how warm-down sets can be used to monitor strength and muscle gains.

Locking your head into a *reasonable* set-rep scheme can rob you of training *passion*. Keep in mind three things. One, plan your workouts. Two, give yourself a rep number to aim at for each set. And three, keep in mind your rep range but seek to overcome it to continually make improvements in your training intensity to effect change to your body.

The point is to not become preoccupied with stopping at a predetermined number of repetitions. This will only slow down your progress or stagnate it. If you can physically and mentally do more, then do more!

Unconventional Rep Range

When I train for muscular endurance my rep range can vary from 20 to 60 reps per set depending on *which* muscle group I am training, *what* technique I am using (e.g., burnsets, dropsets) and *how* I am performing my reps (e.g., full-range, half-range, partial-range, pulsating, static).

I maintain a high rep range when I train small muscles like biceps, triceps, and shoulders. For example, when I exercise side shoulders I sit on a bench and use 5-pound dumbbells (weight is just a measure of resistance how the reps are performed). I perform half reps from mid to top range of motion with a pause at the top for 30 reps, and follow up with pulsating reps at mid-range for 30 reps for a total of 60 reps. Side shoulders are burning, throbbing and swollen.

Next, I train my front shoulders. I sit on a bench and perform either heavy one-arm dumbbell front raises for 15 and 20 reps for 2-3 sets or take a 20-pound barbell sitting down and perform half reps from mid to top range of motion with a pause at the top for 30 reps. Then, without rest, I stand up and perform the same bottom to mid-range for 30 reps. It's short and sweet and gets the job done.

Larger muscle groups can accommodate heavier weight with fewer reps. For chest and lats, I maintain a 30-15 rep range (reverse pyramid). For quadriceps, along with the hips and lower back, I maintain a lower rep range, say 20-10 reps because they are among the biggest and strongest muscle groups in the body with "hidden reserves." Studies have shown that intense leg workouts boost testosterone levels and accelerate fat loss.

Warming-Up and Warm-Up Intensity

A warm-up does four things to the body: (1) increases blood flow to the muscles, which enhances strength, (2) increases flexibility, (3) decreases chance of injury and, (4) foreordains the mindset to establish the mind-body connection for hard physical training.

Warming-up and warm-up intensity go hand-in-hand. No laxing on these. Warming-up does not mean take it easy. It means building your mind and body up for what lies ahead. You should break a sweat during your warm-up. At best you should be breathing heavy.

When you are doing upper body first in your workout and if your gym has an arm cranker, I suggest you use this for 5 to 10-minutes to increase blood flow in the chest, shoulders, biceps, triceps, back and core.

If your gym does not have an arm cranker, then I suggest you start your warm-up with dumbbell shoulder presses for 20 reps. After that, do dumbbell flys for about 15 reps. Finally, continue warming-up on your first exercise, say the bench press for example, using the conventional pyramid scheme 10, 8, 6 to practice good form and to get your head into the game.

Now you are ready and warmed up. Put on the weight and begin your first and heaviest set for as many reps as you can do!

When you do quads first in your workout and squats second after leg extensions (pre-exhaust) I suggest the following warm-up. First, hop on an upright bike. Start peddling and set a resistance level that is challenging for an objective to cycle 3 miles in 8 to 10 minutes at 15 mph for a constant steady-state of 80-85%. When you hop off the bike your quads should be tight and pumped.

Next, and as an option, wrap you knees. Knee wraps can protect your ligaments and joints when lifting intensely. Mr. Blood and Guts himself, Dorian Yates, says he always wrapped his knees before he trained his quads, and to this day claims he has no knee issues because of it.

After that, hop on the leg extension machine and do three to four warm-up back-to-back sets in a controlled mid-range of motion for 15-8 reps using the ascending pyramid weight scheme.

Doing leg extensions first (a single-joint or isolation exercise) before squats or leg presses (a multiple-joint or compound exercise) is a good option before doing squats because extensions not only warm-up the knee joint but it also pre-exhausts the quad muscles.

After your initial 3-4 set warm-up on leg extensions select your weight for your first heaviest set and do 15 or more reps in a controlled fashion with a flex/pause at the top until you can only perform partials to controlled failure. Rest 30 seconds and decrease the weight and do one or two more sets (depending on the routine you are following) in the same manner.

Pre-exhausting the quads with extensions first will enhance the assurance that when you perform a compound movement next like squats it will be safer and harder, yet surprisingly you'll be strong and confident. Lee Haney and Dorian Yates always did leg extensions first before doing squats or leg presses.

Your next exercise is squats. If you need to wear a lifting belt then put one on. Make sure that it as tight as possible. Start with your first heaviest set and do 10 or more non-stop reps. (If you need to do an initial set or two to warm-up for the squat motion, then do it.) Rest long enough to get your breath back before removing a plate for your next set. Gather yourself. Stay focused. Go back under the bar and do one or two more sets in reverse pyramid fashion.

A second warm-up alternative to the one above when you are doing heavy squats first and leg extensions second, I suggest the following.

First, hop on an upright bike. Maintain the same intensity as described above for 8-10 minutes. Second, jump on the leg extension machine. Don't go too heavy as this is still a warm-up for squats. You can train in a rhythmic fashion but not too fast. Extend with a flex/pause. Do 3 sets of 20, 15, 10 in ascending pyramid fashion for 5-10 minutes. And last, go to the squat rack. Do 5 warm-up sets before your first real (and heavy) set.

First, squat with the bar for 20 reps. Second, put a plate on and squat 15 reps. Third, put some more weight on and squat for 10 reps.

Fourth, put additional weight on and squat for 8 reps. And for the last and final warm-up set place more weight on the bar and squat for 2-4 reps. This squat warm-up takes about 10 minutes.

The total warm-up before you actually do your first real set of squats should take 30 minutes. Your mind is ready. Your body is ready. Your joints and tendons are ready. You have established the mind-body connection. You've got this! Now reverse pyramid your way to fitness!

Summary

Does reverse pyramid training work for me? Yes, it does. Will it work for you? Yes, it will. If you want to gain strength quicker, it works. If you want to build muscle quicker, it works. If you want to lose fat quicker, it works. If you want to increase your cardiorespiratory endurance quicker, it works. If you want to get the best buck for your time, it works.

The problem is that most people do not want to take the time to do the initial warm-up that reverse pyramid training demands. But it has been shown in literature how warming-up enhances performance. Reverse pyramid training is not only for the beginner and intermediate but also for the advanced athlete, whatever your health, fitness or professional goal may be.

Reverse pyramid training can help you achieve maximum results in the least amount of time. Reverse pyramid shows you how to: (1) shorten your training time to make it more efficient and productive, (2) expand your knowledge on recuperation and performance nutrition, and (3) train hard, not long.

Habit #6

Train Hard, Not Long to Stimulate Change Quicker

CHAPTER 7

SAME WORKOUTS GET RESULTS

Subject the body to a sufficient amount of stress performing the same workout so that the body can go through the adaptation *process and physiologically change.*

To understand why we *can* get results by doing the *same workout* we must first understand a physiological phenomenon called *'adaptation'*. Why some people get results while others do not is a consequence of the adaptation process.

Preliminary Words

There can be hidden factors why a person does not get results such as having a physiological predisposition. However, before one blames his or her body as the *way it is* as an excuse for not getting results from exercise one must first rule out the adaptation process. But this would be difficult to do if one truly follows the principles of physical fitness and exercises well.

Our bodies are essentially potential energy with a limitless mind only latent to actualize that energy by sharpening our focus with more deliberate and purposeful movement. It is *your* focus, *your* amount of energy, *your* amount of strength, and *your* amount of effort that produces *your* results!

Changing Up Your Routine

Do not "change up" your routine if you think you reached a *'plateau.'* By routine I mean a 3-day a week full-body routine, 4-day a week split routine, or a 5 to 6-day a week split routine. The routine isn't broke. What might be broke is what you think you know or don't know about adaptation.

If you change up your routine prematurely, then your body cannot adapt to the physical stress and change. I stay with the same routine for months or even years because I get results. If I change anything in my routine I will: (1) change the order of exercises, (2) perform a different exercise and (3) incorporate a training technique to train harder with lighter weight.

What is Adaptation?

Adaptation is a process by which the body accustoms itself to physical stress. A certain amount of stress is good for the body. In life, the right amount of stress caused by outside stimuli enables one to progress in whatever one wants to advance in by the means of accustoming oneself to the stress in order to adapt and achieve favorable results.

The gym or your exercise environment is where the body learns the adaptive process, however, on condition that the body is stimulated by exercise stress caused by the exerciser so the body can be superimposed to change its physiological efficiency (inside) and form of composition (outside). That is to say, *to get energy, you must put out energy to get more in return.* Results are invariably linked to effort output and the amount of energy returned.

Three things must occur in the following order for a physiological change to occur:

1. Stress must be stimulated (what you must do)
2. Adaptation is learned (what the body does as a reaction to stress)
3. Change is activated (what happens to the body when stress is applied and adaptation occurs)

When a sufficient amount of exercise stress is stimulated (1), the body reacts by learning to adapt to the stress (2), but if and only if a sufficient amount of stress is applied (1). Change (3) is a consequence of the body adapting (2) to stress (1). In other words, when stress is imposed on the body, the body reacts by learning to adapt to it, which in turn activates change in performance and appearance.

Physiological change cannot take place first without proper stimulation of stress, which in turn follows an adaptive response from the body. This is indeed positive because the body learns from what you have habitually been doing well or what you have become well at doing. The following sequence of events cannot be overemphasized enough:

Stress stimulates → *Body adapts* → *Change occurs*

The "Training Effect"

If there is a significant amount of stress imposed on the body it will invariably undergo a change as a reaction to the stress placed upon it. A constant increase in exercise stress (energy output) to the body leads to strength increases, which causes a change (an increase) in functional ability.

Hence, the body undergoes not one adaptation phase but many. How many adaptations depends on the level of intensity by the amount of energy that is forced on the body at each same workout.

Functional changes in the body are caused by what is called the *Training Effect*. The Training Effect is the body's way of adapting or accustoming itself to physical stress. What follows from the Training Effect are improvements in neuromuscular function (increased strength), cardiorespiratory function (increased endurance), and hypertrophy (increased muscle).

Adaptation and "Reaching a Plateau"

Improving the body is a process and is never-ending. Improvements gradually begin to slow down until the body reaches its limit of adaptation.

When the body reaches its limit from going through consecutive adaptation phases one may be said to have reached a plateau. But "reaching a plateau" has *nothing* to do with repeating the *same workout routine*. The routine does not need fixing. Think again and re-evaluate how comfortable or complacent you might have gotten in your training. Are you motivated? Do you have a loss of energy? Have your flow experiences diminished? Are you in fact *exercising?*

If someone claims to have "reached a plateau" but has *not* gone through many adaptation phases due to a lack of "new stress stimulus" on the body to adapt, then one has *not* reached a plateau.

A plateau is when the body becomes stubborn to adapt and, therefore, change, despite the heightened level of intensity in regard to a change in training weight, system, method or technique. If you think you have reached a plateau because you are not getting results think again. Evaluate your training on two criteria:

1. Effort
2. Adaptation

Systematic Progression for Constant Adaptation

To ensure that the body keeps adapting to the stress imposed upon it in your workouts a "systematic progression" of training needs to be devised that measures the increases in your workout intensity. The best way to measure workout intensity is to do the same exercise but making it harder to do. Keep track of this in a training journal so that you can actually see your own day-to-day and month-to-month progress.

There are several things you can do in your cardio and weight training routines to measure workout intensity and notice a higher level of energy output.

Consider that you have been doing the bike first for 10 minutes in a 60-minute cardio session. You have been at resistance level 12 for quite some time while cycling at 90 revolutions per minute (RPM).

Suppose your goal has been to complete one mile in under 3 minutes or 3 miles under 9 minutes but you have not been able to do this. The reason why this goal has not been achieved is that most likely you have become comfortable cycling at the same level and RPMs and, in effect, have *not* stressed the body enough to adapt in order for change to occur. But now is the time for the body to adapt to a new level of stress.

Increase the bike resistance level to 13 and speed to 95RPM. When your mind starts to fatigue say to yourself, "Be one with the machine. Mold yourself into it. Work with it." Get into the flow of exercising. Your mind will become stronger and you will be able to maintain a constant steady-state of 80-85% until you are done.

You will discover that only after a few workouts with this particular cardio exercise at this new level of resistance and RPM that your goal time is achievable. These small changes in workout intensity can be sustainable due to an increase in strength and cardiorespiratory endurance.

Another consideration is the stairmill. Suppose you have been doing speed level 8 for quite some time for 10 minutes and holding on the entire time (i.e., holding on and upright and not leaning forward by putting your own weight on the bar handles).

Suppose your goal is do the stairmill without holding on for the entire 10 minutes. Slowly and systematically work up to this goal.

Begin by holding on for the first 9 minutes but let go the last minute. It is harder doing the stairmill while you are not holding on. The next time you do the stairmill hold on for the first 8 minutes but let go the last two minutes, and so on until you are not holding on for the entire 10 minutes!

This is how you can see and measure an increase in your workout intensity and notice changes to the body. The body is forced to adapt to the constant increase of stress and noticeable increases in strength, muscle, endurance, balance and coordination can be experienced because of a stronger mind. A stronger mind means more intense workouts, more adaptations and continual changes to the body.

Consider measuring intensity in your weight training by making a set harder to complete on a particular exercise using a controlled technique.

Suppose you have mastered doing dumbbell flys with a weight in great form with 15 reps. The eccentric movement is controlled, your elbows are slightly bent with arms out, your concentric movement is strong and you stop a foot's length between each dumbbell at the top of the movement for constant tension. But now is the time for the body to adapt to a new level of stress.

To create more tension in the pectoral muscles, use the same weight and form. However, when performing the eccentric movement pause the weight at the bottom (where the stress is greatest and the potential for more muscle growth) for 1-2 seconds before performing the concentric movement. This forces more stress on the outer pecs and teaches you to use your mind more because of the greater tension you will feel. Remember the "time under tension" principle.

The last thing you might consider is to invest in a heart rate technology so you can see where your heart rate is at and work up to maintaining a constant steady-state of 80-85%. I discovered that when I used a certain heart rate technology in my training, I burned over 800 calories during my cardio routine and over 900 during my weight routine in less than one hour.

The Same Workout and Adaptation

Instead of changing up your routine frequently to "confuse the body" by reading training articles by advanced athletes I offer this suggestion: Subject your body to the same workout routine for months or even a year to maximize the Training Effect by mastering the movement of each particular exercise to exercise well.

Maximizing the Training Effect can only be accomplished by triggering maximal "specific adaptations" with the same workout for a period length of time.

Why Adaptation Does Not Occur

It is most likely that unexperienced exercise enthusiasts have never even come close to exercise adaptation to qualify for reaching a plateau. There are four reasons why:

1. A lack of exercise effort and, therefore, exercise stress.
2. Confusing work with exercise.
3. A lack of high-performance nutrition.
4. Adherence to an unsuitable training routine or none at all.

Subjecting oneself to the same workout gives appreciation to both the mind and body working together. Since the mind controls the body and the body obeys the mind the same workout can develop into a higher level of intensity to stimulate stress and force the body to adapt and change composition and increase functional ability.

Habit #7

Perform the Same Workout Routine to Undergo Many Adaptation Phases

CHAPTER 8

―――――――――

EXERCISING MORE EFFECTIVELY

When you know how *the limbs on your body move and* how *the muscles function in relation to that movement and joint alignment with other joints can make an exercise safe and effective, then you can train intelligently and get results.*

Exercising more effectively is understanding the planes of motion, joint movement, muscle function, and joint alignment.

Three Planes of Motion

Three basic reference planes are used in kinesiology of motion: (1) sagittal plane, (2) frontal or coronal plane, and (3) transverse plane.[86, 87] A muscle is responsible for moving a limb or limbs in each plane of motion at a joint. Muscles can have more than one function and involve more than one plane of motion. And some muscles rely on the function of other muscles to move them apart from the joint they specifically move.[88]

Each plane of motion with exercises involved will be explained and described first before proceeding to the next plane and exercises.[89] But first, two terms need to be defined, namely, *flexion* and *extension*.

On the one hand, flexion means decreasing the angle between two joints. When an elbow flexion movement is performed by flexing the biceps you are bringing the hand closer to the shoulder and, thus, *shortening* the angle between the shoulder and elbow joint. On the other hand, extension means increasing the angle between two joints. When an elbow extension movement is performed by extending the triceps you are taking the hand further away from the shoulder and, thus, *lengthening* the angle between the shoulder and elbow joint.

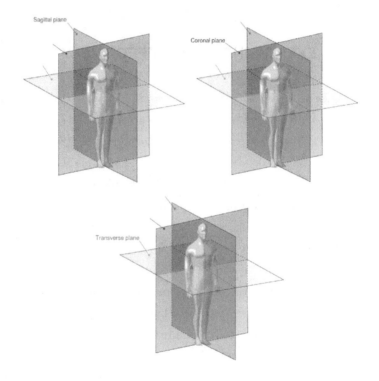

Describing each plane of motion with the muscles and exercises involved, first, I state each plane of motion in the direction connected to the moving limbs of the body. Next, I describe a muscle function related to its plane of motion and joint movement. Then, I mention an exercise or two associated with its plane of motion. After that, I detail the joint alignment and body position of the said exercise.[90] And finally, I explain the ROM of each exercise along with some noteworthy suggestions.[91]

Sagittal Plane of Motion

The sagittal plane cuts the body into right and left halves. Motion in the sagittal plane moves *up and down or forward and backward with the body*. Every muscle in the sagittal plane is exhausted: chest, shoulders, biceps, triceps, back, low back, quadriceps, hamstrings, calves, and abdominals.

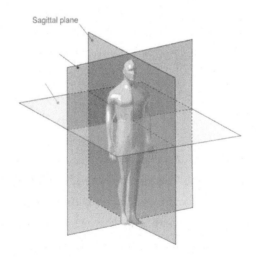

Most exercises take place in the sagittal plane: chest dips, chest pullovers, shoulder presses, shoulder front raises, biceps curls, triceps pushdowns, pulldowns, bent-over rows, deadlifts, back squats, leg extensions, hamstring curls, calf raises, walking, running, climbing stairs, arm cranking, the rope trainer, and battle ropes.

Chest Muscle and Exercises

Chest Function. Responsible for moving the upper limbs (arms) up and toward the midline of the body by "flexing" the shoulder joint from a vertical to horizontal position from the floor. Exercises include chest dips and chest pullovers.

Chest Dips: Joint Alignment and Body Position. Elbows bent and facing back and away from the midline of the body with wrists. Elbows and shoulder joints are in alignment.

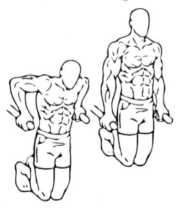

Chest Dips ROM. Preferably shoulder width if bars allow. Lean forward a bit to emphasize the chest muscles.[92] Start with elbows slightly bent. Dip down by bending the elbows and stop when the upper arms are horizontal to the floor or slightly below. Push up and stop with elbows slightly bent before repeating the movement.

Chest Pullovers: Joint Alignment and Body Position. Lie down on a flat bench. A flat bench stabilizes the whole body and keeps the motion strong and safe rather than lying sideways with the upper back across a bench. Take a shoulder width grip if you are using a crooked (not straight) bar. If you are using a dumbbell, clasp the dumbbell with the palms of your hands with one over the other. The dumbbell should be in alignment with the head rather than the shoulders. The elbows are slightly bent throughout the motion and facing up and forward and toward the midline of the body with wrists, elbows and shoulders in alignment.

Chest Pullovers ROM. With elbows slightly bent, lower the resistance down and above the head and back (bottom drawing first). Stop when the arms are slightly above horizontal to the floor. Push the weight back up above your head and stop preferably at a 60-degree angle for constant tension before repeating the movement. Do not lockout the elbows to support the weight with the elbow joints. This can lead to an injury.

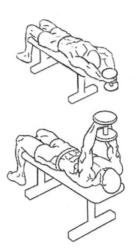

Front Shoulder Muscle and Exercises

Front Shoulder Function. Responsible for moving the arms up and away from the midline of the body by "extending" the shoulder joint. Exercises include shoulder presses and front raises. Sit on a bench with a back support for safety, stability, and strength (unlike the drawing).

Shoulder Press: Joint Alignment and Body Position. Hand placement is wider than shoulder width. The elbows are out and away from the midline of the body. *Barbell:* wrists, elbows, and shoulder joints are in alignment. Forearms are vertical to the floor. *Dumbbells:* wrists, elbows, and shoulder joints are *not* in alignment to prevent unnecessary shoulder joint stress. Forearms are vertically offset from the floor toward the body. In other words, move the wrists in a few inches toward the body by bending the elbow joint in slightly.

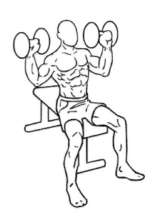

Shoulder Press ROM. If you are using a barbell and starting overhead, lower the bar in front of the head until the bar meets your chin or below to the neck. Push the weight up and back. Stop before locking out the elbows. If you are using dumbbells, push the weight up and in toward the body and overhead, but don't clang the dumbbells together. Lower the weight back down until the dumbbells are in alignment with the ears and upper arms are below horizontal to the floor.

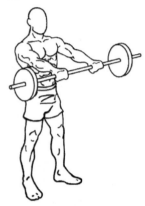

Front Raise: Joint Alignment and Body Position. Elbows are out and away from the midline of the body and slightly bent. Front raises can either be performed using dumbbells or a straight or crooked barbell. Front raises can also be performed either using a supinated (palms up and elbows down), pronated (palms down and elbows out) or neutral (palms facing each other) grip with a slight supination. A neutral grip can only be performed with dumbbells. In all cases, the thumb is preferably placed on the outside of the handles or bar to prevent forearm assistance when raising the weight up.

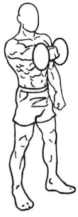

Whether you choose a barbell or dumbbell the hand placement is *not* in alignment with the shoulder joint but approximately six inches away from it. Placing the arms slightly angled out (for all raise movements) and away from the midline of the body can prevent a minor function of the chest occurring, which is to elevate or raise the shoulder.

Front Raise ROM. Barbell or dumbbell front raises can either be performed seated or standing. Start approximately 8-12 inches away from the body to prevent momentum. Lean forward at the hips a bit to prevent assistance from the traps to help raise the weight. Raise the weight using the front shoulders while doing your best to deactivate the traps by retracting and depressing the shoulder blades (scapula) with the lat muscles.[93] Stop when the weight is horizontal to the floor. Hold the upward position for a second. Lower the weight 8-12 inches from the body and repeat.

Bicep Muscle and Exercise

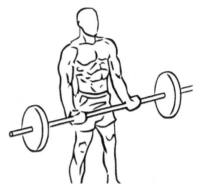

Biceps Function. The biceps are composed of two muscles and are smaller than the triceps. Responsible for moving the lower limb (forearm) up toward the shoulder by "flexing" the elbow joint and rotating the forearm by turning the palm upward (supination).[94] For this reason, barbell curls with a straight bar is preferred. Position variations: standing, seated, kneeling, lying, bent-over, elbows down, elbows up. Exercises include all bicep elbow flexion movements. A basic exercise is standing biceps curl.

Standing Biceps Curls: Joint Alignment and Body Position. Take a supinated grip on the bar with thumbs on the inside and wrist straight (unlike the drawing). Arms are near vertical to the floor, slightly forward. Elbows face back and toward the midline of the body. The wrist, elbow, and shoulder are all in alignment. Shoulder blades are retracted and the knees are slightly bent.

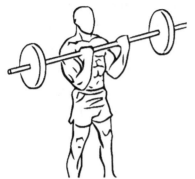

Standing Biceps Curls ROM. "Pull" the weight up while maintaining proper joint alignment. The movement stops with the angle of the forearms and hands/wrists 45 degrees from the shoulders.[95] This is a complete elbow flex position for the biceps without making the mistake of going past this angle by "excessively" leaning back and pulling the weight forward and flexing the shoulder joint (like the drawing; don't do this). Consciously flex or squeeze the biceps at this 45-degree stopping point. Lower the weight back down to the start position with elbows slightly bent and repeat. Locking out the elbows will "take away" the muscle tension.

Tricep Muscle and Exercise

Triceps Function. The triceps are composed of three muscles and are larger than the biceps. Responsible for moving the lower limb (forearm) down by "extending" the elbow joint to a locked position for a full

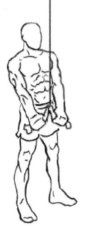

contraction and vertical to the floor. A basic exercise is standing cable triceps pushdowns.

Tricep Pushdowns: Joint Alignment and Body Position. The movement starts with the elbows bent and upper arms vertical to the floor. Take a pronated grip with thumbs over the upside down "V" shape bar. The hands are approximately 60 degrees from the shoulders. Elbows face down and toward the midline of the body. The wrist, elbow, and shoulder are all in alignment. Lean forward at the hips, arch the lower back, stick out the butt, retract the shoulder blades, lift up the chest, and bend your knees slightly (unlike the drawing). This positioning helps to stabilize the whole upper body and alleviate lower back, shoulder, and elbow joint strain.

Triceps Pushdowns ROM. Once again, start 60 degrees from the shoulders. "Push" down the resistance until the elbows are in a fully locked and extended position and repeat.

Back (lat) Muscle and Exercises

Lat Function. Responsible for moving the upper limbs (arms) down and toward the midline of the body by "flexing" the shoulder joint and pulling in or retracting the shoulder blades (scapula). This exercise promotes spinal stability and better posture. Exercises include seated lat pulldowns and bent-over dumbbell rows.[96]

Lat Pulldowns: Joint Alignment and Body Position. Take a wider than shoulder width grip with a pronated grip, thumb over the bar and elbows pointed down (unlike the drawing).[97] Imagine your fingers as hooks on the bar and your arms as extensions of the hooks. Pulling down in this manner will alleviate forearm and upper arm assistance.

Sit down, lift up the chest, arch the back, and lean back by extending at the hips to a 20 to 30-

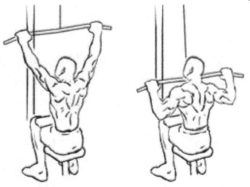

degree angle (unlike the drawing). "Pull" the bar down and towards the body to the throat with elbows pointing down and forward (unlike the drawing). The wrists and elbows should be in alignment and in the same 20 to 30-degree angle with the upper body.[98]

Lat Pulldowns ROM. Pull the bar down at an angle so that it is directly in front of your throat. As you pull down, consciously bring the elbows in toward the sides of the body. "Jab" the elbows to the sides of the body and pull in (retract) the shoulder blades to the midline of the body. ROM should stop where the bar is directly in front of your throat (not above or below chest) to where you cannot physically retract the blades any further. Resist the weight up without rocking forward to keep muscle tension on the lats.

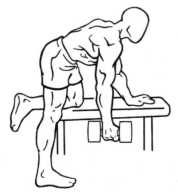

Bent-Over Dumbbell Rows: Joint Alignment and Body Position. Whether you place the palm of your hand on another dumbbell on the rack, place the palm of your hand on top of a 45-degree angle incline bench or place a bent knee and palm of your hand on a flat bench to support the body position for rows it doesn't matter. What matters is your preference. I will describe the latter position on a flat bench and perform dumbbell rows on the right side of the body (like the drawing).

Place the left bent knee and lower leg limb (shin) on a bench with the ankle hanging over the side of the bench. Extend the right leg out alongside the bench with a bent knee to support upper body and core stability.

Place the left hand in front of the left knee on the bench gripping the front of the bench for stability. Bend or flex the hips to lower the upper body into position (like the drawing). Lift up the chest, arch the lower back, stick out your glutes, and lower the hips down a bit toward the bench.

Bent-Over Dumbbell Rows ROM. Pick up the dumbbell off the floor with a neutral grip and thumb over the handle. "Hook" the fingers around the handle. "Pull" the weight up and back toward the midline of the body with elbow in. The upper arm and forearm are approximately 90-degrees (like the drawing).

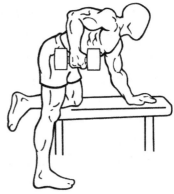

In this top and completed position, retract the right shoulder blade while keeping both hips and shoulders in alignment without "twisting" the spine (this is the transverse plane) in order to retain a straight and flat (not rounded) back. When this exercise is performed properly the oblique muscles may be sore the next day because of the "static" position to help stabilize the movement while lifting on one side of the body.

Lower Back (Lumbar Spine) and Exercise

Lower Back (Lumbar Spine). The lower back is made up the erector spinae and gluteal muscles. Exercises for this region include "hip-hinge" movements, such as, deadlifts, back extensions, and good mornings. Other muscles involved in exercising the lower back that involve the "hip-hinge" movement include: quadriceps, hamstrings, abdominals and rhomboids. Let's briefly go over these muscle functions first and then take a look at deadlifts.

Erector Spinae function. Responsible for straightening (neutral position) and rotating the back.[99]

Glute function. Responsible for extending (upward motion) the spine and knees at the hip joint. The gluteal muscles are also responsible for moving toward the midline of the body (the crack) by flexing the butt cheeks (upward motion).

Quadriceps function. Responsible for extending the knee away from the midline of the body (upward deadlift motion) and flexing the hips toward the midline of the body (downward deadlift motion).

Hamstring function. Responsible for flexing the knee toward the midline of the body (downward deadlift motion). Think of the hamstrings as the "braking" muscle when the weight is slowly being lowered to the floor.

Abdominals function. Responsible for strengthening and stabilizing the core.

Rhomboid function. Responsible for pulling in (retracting) the shoulder blades (upward and downward deadlift motion).

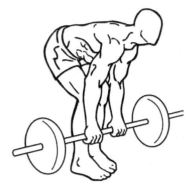

Deadlifts: Joint Alignment and Body Position. Take a hip width stance and place the feet under the bar with the bar near the shins. Take an overhand/underhand grip (unlike the drawing) and shoulder width grip on the bar on the outside of the thighs.[100] Bend the knees to get into a squat position and drive your hips down and back to the floor. Lift up the chest and retract the shoulder blades to activate the erector spinae muscles for a neutral spine position.

All of the joints in this start position should be in alignment from your feet, ankles, knees, hips, shoulders, elbows, and wrists. The back is neutral, straight, and flat. *Do not* begin this great exercise in a curved spine (back flexion) position!

Deadlifts ROM. Plant your heels, sit back, retract the shoulder blades, lift up the chest, drive the glutes and hips down and "pull!" Use the quadriceps to extend the knee back and extend the hips forward. Continue to drive the hips forward by squeezing the glutes to stand erect.

Keep retracting the shoulder blades while resisting the weight downward to the floor with the hamstrings and hips, but don't drop the weight. You are only as strong as your "negative" repetition. Most injuries occur during the downward (negative) motion of a repetition. Either "reset" the weight and re-grip or "tap it" on the floor before repeating.

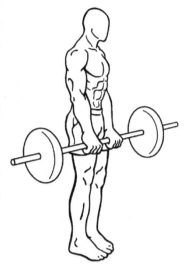

Quadricep Muscles and Exercises

Quadriceps Function. The "quads" are composed of four muscles. Responsible for flexing the hip joint toward the midline of the body and extending the knee joint away from the midline of the body. Exercises include back squats and leg extensions. Other muscles involved in performing the back squat that involve the "hip-hinge" movement include: erector spinae, hamstrings, glutes, abdominals and rhomboids. Let's go over these muscles briefly and see how they function in the squat before taking a look at barbell back squats.

Erector Spinae function. Responsible for straightening and rotating the back. This muscle keeps your back straight and flat and in a neutral spine position.

Hamstring function. Responsible for flexing the knee toward the midline of the body (downward squat motion). This is the "braking" muscle again while descending into a squat position.

Glute function. Responsible for extending the hips and knees forward away from the midline of the body (upward squat motion). Technically, the glutes do not have a function when performing squats. But they do have a benefit. During the eccentric (downward) squat motion the glute muscles stretch (lengthen) as to why you might feel a "butt burn" either doing squats or leg presses, especially when performing high repetitions.

Abdominals function. Responsible for strengthening and stabilizing the core.

Rhomboid function. Responsible for pulling in (retracting) the shoulder blades (upward and downward squat motion).

Barbell Back Squats: Joint Alignment and Body Position. Place the bar on the back of the traps above the rear shoulders and your hands anywhere on the bar between your body and the rack hooks. If you have tight elbow tendons and shoulders you might want to grasp the bar all the way out to the ends of each side after you remove it from the rack.

Remove the weight off the rack and take a few steps back to take your preferred feet width stance. I prefer a hip width feet position. Feet placement can be a personal preference for a safe, secure, strong and effective squat. Feet width position is important because it has been said that you should "never let your knees go past your toes while doing a squat." The reasoning for this is to avoid excessive forward movement of the knees over the toes during a squat movement. But is there merit to this advice? Yes and no. It is a *myth* that you should "never let your knees go past your toes while doing a squat." This belief originated from a study 40 years ago in the late 70s. The fact is that learning forward too much is more likely to cause an injury and not the exercise itself.[101]

As an ectomorph, I biomechanically have long limbs and a short upper body. My limbs travel far to get into a full squat position. So, I have to work harder than a person who is more balanced. But squats have been my favorite next to deadlifts. I've been squatting for over 40 years with my knees going past my toes, but I have no knee issues. It depends on where the force of the weight is placed.

Keep the heels planted on the floor during a squat motion. You'll be pushing your heels into the floor going down and also pushing up off the floor with your heels to prevent your toes from doing the pushing. This is the trick and the secret to squatting. Planting the heels on the floor can help distribute the weight back and not forward. Lift up the chest to activate the abs and erector spinae muscles to get into a neutral spine position (straight and flat). Slowly descend into a squat hip flexion position as you work the hamstrings flexing at the knee joint. *Back Squats ROM.* Descend into a parallel or slightly above parallel position without breaking the kinetic chain feet, ankles, knees and hips alignment. "Push" the weight back up by driving your upper body up and back while extending the hips and knees forward to an "unlocked" position to maintain tension and a neutral spine and repeat.[102]

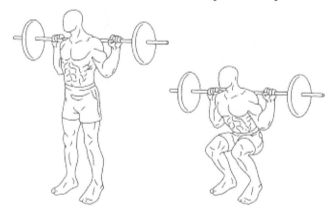

When performing a squat from start to finish it is important to track the knees over toes to prevent them from turning inward or "caving in." This caving in of the knees is most likely due to weak abductor muscles on the lateral or side of the leg, which can break a strong kinetic chain of motion. If this happens correct it because it can lead to a knee injury. At best, focus on keeping the knees open. The feet, ankles, knees and hips should all be in alignment.

Leg Extensions: Joint Alignment and Body Position. Before you sit down on the machine select the weight and adjust the shin pad to the length of your legs. Sit down on the machine and place the shins underneath the pad. Adjust the seat so the lower back is in contact with the back support and the back of the knees are flush against the front part of the seat. Sit down and grab a hold of the handles and start extending the knee out and away from the body while keeping the toes, shins, knees and hips in alignment. Do not use high-impact fast jerky movements as this can lead to a knee injury.[103]

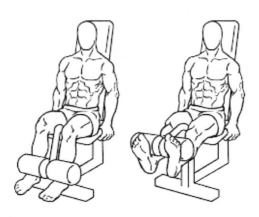

Leg Extensions ROM. Relax the shins under the pad by pointing the toes down (not up). This will transfer the weight onto the quadriceps rather than feeling it in the knees. Pointing the toes up toward the body by extending the ankle will transfer some of the weight onto the knees. Use the lower limbs (legs) to extend the knees out and away from the body by using the powerful quadricep muscles. Fully extend the knees and lockout. Consciously hold the contracted position for a pause-flex-squeeze. Lower to start position slowly, but do not go down all the way where you lose tension in the quadriceps. Stop with the knees still extending out and lower limbs away from the machine to ensure constant tension throughout the set.

Many people hate doing leg extensions because it produces an unbearable burn in the quad muscles. But, as already mentioned above, this "burn" is due to reduced blood flow to the muscle. As a consequence of the burn, people prematurely stop the exercise long before the muscles actually fatigue because of pain signals sent to the brain by the spine. But certain parts of the brain stem can inhibit incoming pain signals by the production of endorphins and block the pain, which allows one to keep exercising through the burn. The challenge is to train consistency and with the same approximate intensity in order to mentally build up the endurance to train in the burn zone until the burn subsides and the muscles physically fatigue to the point of failure. The more consistent and constant you are with your training and intensity the body will adapt to the burning sensation and will eventually lessen.

Hamstring Muscles and Exercise

Hamstring Function. The hamstrings are composed of three long muscles. Responsible for flexing the knee toward the midline of the body (up or downward motion of leg curls). Exercises include lying leg curls, seated leg curls, standing one-leg curls, and stiff-leg deadlifts. Let's take a look at lying leg curls.[104]

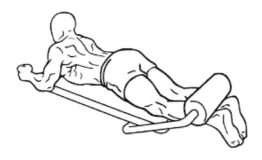

Lying Leg Curls: Joint Alignment and Body Position. Before lying face down on the machine adjust the ankle pad to the length of your legs. Select the weight, lie down, position the ankles under the pad with the toes pointing down and toward the body. Grab a hold of the handles.

Keep the neck and shoulders down to alleviate tenson in the neck and lower back (unlike the drawing). *Lying Leg Curls ROM.* Flex or bend the knee joint and curl the pad up to the butt while keeping the toes, ankles, knees and hips n alignment. Return the ankle pad to a slightly bent knee starting position. Do not fully extend the knee joint.

Calf Muscles and Exercises

Calf Function. Responsible for flexing the ankle joint by pointing the foot and toes downward. Exercises include machine standing calf raises and plate loaded seated calf raises (one of my favorites). One leg standing calf raises is an excellent option for working the calf muscles.

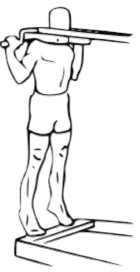

Standing Calf Raises: Joint Alignment and Body Position. This exercise primarily works the gastrocnemius muscle. Place the toes of the feet on an elevated platform. Bend the knees slightly to alleviate unnecessary tension off the hamstrings and achilles tendon. Push up off the toes and flex the calf muscles while keeping the toes, ankles, knees and hips in alignment. Descend by extending the heels of the feet down toward the floor to lengthen the calf muscle.

Standing Calf Raises ROM. Select your desired resistance. Place your traps under the pads and hands on the handles or in front. Push up off the toes and contract the calf muscles while depressing the traps.[105] Hold this position for two seconds and return slowly to starting position where the heel is pointing down toward the floor. Hold this position for one second and repeat.

Seated Calf Raises: Joint Alignment and Body Position. This exercise works both the gastrocnemius and soleus muscles. This is a great exercise for strengthening the ankles for sports like gymnastics, ice skating, and soccer. Sit down and adjust the knee pads to the point where they are very snug against the top of the lower thighs above the knees. Position the feet and toes on the platform with the toes, ankles and knees in alignment.

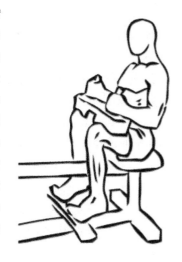

Seated Calf Raises ROM. Place on your desired weight. Grasp the vertical hand grips and push the toes up off the platform. Flex the calf muscles and pause at the top of the movement. Keep your upper body strong and tight like the drawing and not leaning forward or hunched over while sitting. Return for a full stretch and repeat.

Abdominal Muscles and Exercises[106]

Abdominal (Lower, Oblique, Upper) Function. Because the abdominal muscles run vertical to the body, and are relatively short, they are responsible for flexing or rounding the spine (not flexing the hips and extending or arching the lower back) and moving the upper body forward toward the midline of the body requiring only a few inches of movement. In other words, ab training is a "back flexion" movement.

Any abdominal training will require you to already begin in a spinal flexion position. Obviously, the hip flexors will be involved in ab training. But the idea is to keep them to a minimum and focus on back flexion, not hip flexion. Minimizing hip flexion is more difficult to do when performing any leg or knee raise movement to work the abs.

Performing abdominal exercises strengthen and support the lower back, but they do not burn off the fat around the tummy area. Spot reduction is a myth. Exercises include leg raises, oblique leg raise crunches, and abdominal crunches.

A suggestion for ab training is to visualize yourself trying to shorten the distance between the rib cage and pelvis (flexing the hips and arching the back does the opposite). In other words, try to bring the bottom of the rib cage to meet the top of the pelvis. This can ensure the constant tension in only the few inches that it requires. Performing a few inches range of movement for the abs is difficult because of the tendency to flex at the hips more than necessary at the expense of minimizing spinal flexion.

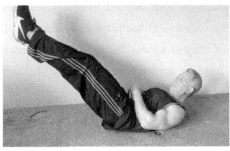

Leg Raise (Lower): Joint Alignment and Body Position. This is a common ab movement. Whether you are doing leg raises lying down on the floor, on an apparatus supporting the upper body and raising the knees to the chest or grasping a bar overhead with the legs dangling below you and raising the knees to the chest, the "back flexion" rule remains the same.

If you are doing these hanging, then I strongly suggest you get into a quarter pullup position to avoid the hips swaying back and forth to stabilize yourself. Tilt the hips forward and up by getting into a spinal flexion position to maximize this motion. This is a challenging exercise.

If you are using an apparatus, then suppress the lower back against the back of the pad and lean the upper body forward by flexing the back. And last, but not least, if you are performing this exercise lying down (pictured on the previous page), then suppress the lower back against the floor and start the movement with the lower legs approximately three feet or more off the floor. This will allow you to get into a spinal flexion position when you start. Starting in this ROM position is similar to reverse crunches. Regardless of which exercise you choose to perform, joint alignment remains the same: ankles, knees and hips while trying to minimize a forward neck.

Leg Raises (Lower) ROM. As stated above, when you do these on the floor start approximately three feet or more off the floor. Lift the shoulder blades up off the floor and always assume this

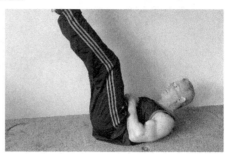

back flexion position. Place the hands and arms across the abs. Pull the legs back and towards the body a few inches by doing your best to flex the spine more than the hips. Return the legs to start position while keeping the shoulder blades up off the floor and repeat.

Oblique (Side) Leg Raise Crunches: Joint Alignment and Body Position. Because the oblique muscles run diagonally down towards the midline of the body, they are trained by rotating *and* flexing the spine. This ab exercise is performed either on a bench or the floor. Performing it on a bench will require you to balance on one side of your body without falling off, which is more challenging. This is my favorite ab exercise. Let's do these on the floor.

Lie down and tilt the whole body to the left side with the left hip positioned on the floor and feet two or more feet off the floor. Elevate your upper body up and off the floor by doing a side rotation back flexion movement. Also, elevate your left shoulder up and off the floor so that you are not using your left arm to stabilize and balance. Your upper body remains stationary throughout the movement as you'll only be moving your legs up and down. You'll be balancing on your left butt while training the right oblique. Now balance. Keep the ankles, thighs and knees together.

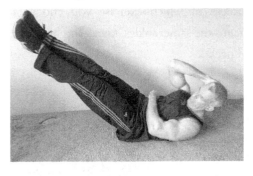

Oblique (Side) Leg Raise Crunches ROM. Once again, the oblique muscles run diagonally down towards the midline of the body. Since you are balancing on your left cheek, take your left hand and place it on the right oblique. Take your right hand and place it behind your head.

The direction of the movement is the right elbow to the right knee. That is the direction (not the ROM) of the movement. Now pull the legs up toward the right side of your body and do your best to shorten the space between your right rib cage and right hip until they meet and "crunch" (end position, pictured). Return your feet to two or more feet off the floor and repeat. Now switch sides.

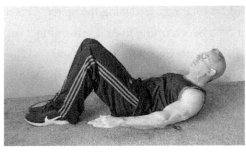

Crunches (Upper): Joint Alignment and Body Position. This simple crunch movement is best performed on the floor. Lie down. Place both feet on the floor with bent knees. The feet, knees and hips are in alignment. Either place the hands behind your head, the arms folded across your chest or the arms to your sides extended straight with palms facing down (pictured). Lift the shoulder blades up off the floor by flexing the back a bit for the start position.

Crunches (Upper) ROM. Pull the upper body up by flexing the spine a few inches more to keep the spine flat on the floor without flexing the hips. Hold the position for a second (pictured) and return to start position while keeping the shoulder blades up off the floor.

Frontal or Coronal Plane of Motion

The frontal/coronal plane cuts the body into front and back halves. Motion in the frontal plane moves *toward or away from the side of the body.* Exercises include: side shoulder raises, side leg raises, and side bends at the waist. Let's look at side shoulder raises.

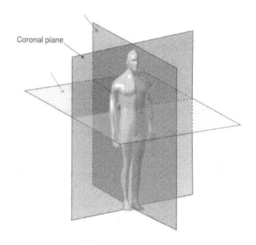

Coronal plane

Side Shoulder Muscles and Exercise

Side Shoulder Raise Function. Responsible for moving the arms up and away from the body and towards the body or away from the body as in horizontal flexion and external rotation.[107] Exercises include any side raise dumbbell movements.

Side Shoulder Raise: Joint Alignment and Body Position. Hold the dumbbells with a pronated grip with thumbs over the handle. Twist the wrists slightly downward so the thumbs are slightly facing down and the elbows slightly bent and facing back and in alignment with the shoulders.

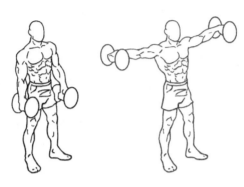

Side Shoulder Raise ROM: Lean forward at the hips to alleviate some trapezius assistance and start the movement 8-12 inches from the body (unlike the drawing). Stop the movement just before the upper arms are horizontal to the floor (unlike the drawing). Hold the top position for a second before returning the weight by keeping it 8-12 inches from the body.

Many people make the mistake of throwing the weight up using the body's momentum to where it breaks horizontal due to the assistance of the trapezius. Then they lower the weight down until it crosses in front of the body in order to build up more momentum. Where's the constant tension? Suggestion: lower the resistance by half or more. The side shoulders are small muscles. They do not require a lot of weight. Start with arms out and away from the body at 8-12 inches. Stop the upward movement before horizontal and pause the position before returning.

Transverse Plane of Motion

The transverse plane cuts the body into top and bottom halves. Motion in the transverse plane moves *toward or away from the midline of the body, including "twisting" or rotation of a limb or the spine.* Exercises include: chest press, chest flys, reverse flys (rear lateral raises), seated hip adduction, abduction machines, hanging twisting leg raises, arm cranking, battle ropes, and rotating the knees, ankles, wrists, waist and neck. I will confine myself to the first three exercises.

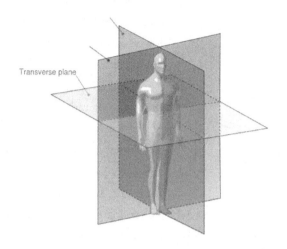

Transverse plane

Chest Muscle and Exercises

Chest Function. Responsible for moving the arms across the body and up and down. Exercises include: chest press with dumbbells and chest flys.

Chest Press: Joint Alignment and Body Position. Elbows are away from the midline of the body and in alignment with the wrist. Elbows are slightly forward to avoid unnecessary strain on the shoulder girdle. That is, the elbows are not in alignment with the shoulders. Hand width for most chest pressing movements is wider than shoulder width with the forearms either vertical to the floor (barbell) or angled in toward the body (dumbbells).

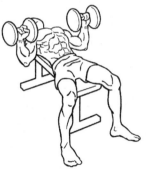

Chest Press ROM. Slowly lower the resistance until the upper arms are below horizontal. Push the resistance back up and stop before locking out the elbows and repeat.

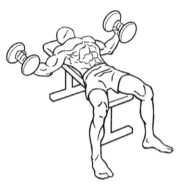

Chest Fly: Joint Alignment and Body Position. Slightly bent elbows with lower arms (forearms) away and angled out from the body. *Chest Dumbbell Fly ROM:* Lower the arms out and away from the body. Stop when the upper arms are horizontal to the floor or slightly below. Pause and hold for one second. Push the weight back up and stop when the hands are at least 8-12 inches apart from one another (unlike the drawing). Do not clang the dumbbells together. If you are using a machine for chest flys the ROM begins in the opposite direction but otherwise the same as described above.

Rear Shoulder Muscles and Exercise

Rear Shoulders Function. Responsible for extending the shoulder joint back and toward the midline of the body. The muscles responsible for moving the rear shoulders back (reverse fly motion) are the *lat* and *rhomboid* muscles. The lat and rhomboid muscles "retract" the rear shoulders by pulling them back toward the midline of the body.

"Protracted" rear shoulders, as well as protracted shoulder blades (rhomboids), account for the *forward posture position* that most people exhibit because of long hours in that position, e.g., sitting at a computer.

Rear pull movements can be done with a variety of exercises either standing in a bent-over position, seated facing forward on a selectorized machine or lying on an incline bench facing down using dumbbells. In all cases, the form and ROM remain the same.

The drawing shows the latter exercise (head supported against a bench, yet not necessary) with generally good form in a horizontal body position, joint alignment, and ROM. I will describe this exercise visually using a selectorized machine facing forward and in a vertical seated position (not bent-over like the drawing) because it is

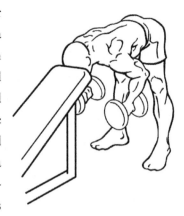

easier and safer to perform, yet the form remains the same as in the drawing.

Rear Shoulders: Joint Alignment and Body Position. Adjust the arms of the machine by moving them in to the first (or last) hole so the horizontal handles are in front of you. Adjust the seat position so the handles are in alignment with the rear shoulders when you sit down. Sit down facing the machine and select a reasonable amount of weight that is not heavy.

Grab the handles with thumbs on the outside and elbows slightly bent and facing back and down. Position the chest against the pad and lift the chest up. Arch the lower back and retract the shoulder blades.

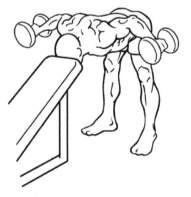

Rear Shoulders ROM: Before you start, consciously depress (relax) the trapezius by lowering the shoulders and consciously pull your neck back to align the ears with the shoulders. Pull the arms of the machine back and away from the sides of your body and extend the shoulder joint back as the lat and rhomboid muscles retract the rear shoulder muscles.

Stop the movement when the upper arms, elbows and shoulder joints are in alignment and not beyond! Return to the start position while keeping your shoulder blades retracted, back arched and chest lifted up. Stop at the start ROM when your hands are approximately two or more feet apart to keep resisting the weight for constant tension.

APPENDICES

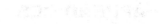

APPENDIX A-1

WEIGHT TRAINING ROUTINE PRE-COVID-19

This is the 3-4 day a week full-body 60-minute weight routine that I frequently use in the gym. I rotate upper or lower body first in my workout every other day. I accommodate myself by doing specific exercises for chest, shoulders, and triceps due to sustained injuries in my mid-50s.

<u>Upper body warm-up</u>: 10 minutes
Arm cranker: resistance level highest; both arms 5 minutes; each arm for 30 second intervals for 5 minutes.

<u>Upper body</u>
Chest (burnsets: 1 & 2)
1. Dumbbell flys 2 x 20
2. Dumbbell pullovers 2 x 20
3. Incline dumbbell landmines 1 x 20-30

Shoulders (burnsets: 4 & 5)
4. Seated barbell front raises (pause at top) 1 x 30
5. Standing barbell front raises (pause at midpoint) 1 x 30
6. Seated dumbbell side raises (mid-range only) 1 x 30

7. Seated rotator cuff exercise 1 x 15

Lats (burnsets)

8. Seated cable rows 20, 15

9. Standing stiff-arm pulldowns 20, 15

Rhomboids & rear shoulders (burnsets)

10. Machine reverse flys; leaning forward, elbows bent 2 x 20

11. Machine reverse flys; upright, elbows slightly bent 2 x 12

Biceps & Triceps (supersets)

12. Barbell curls 3 x 20

13. Assisted or machine dips 3 x 20

Lower body warm-up: 10 minutes

Stationary bike: resistance level 15; distance 3 miles; time 8:30; RPM 90-100.

Lower body

Quads & Lower back (superset)

14. Squats 2 x 12

15. Deadlifts 2 x 12

Hams & Quads (superset)

16. Seated leg curls 3 x 15

17. Leg extensions 2 x 15-20

Calves & Abs (superset)

18. Standing calf raises 3 x 15

19. Knee raises on apparatus 3 x 20

APPENDIX A-2

CARDIO TRAINING ROUTINE PRE-COVID-19

This is a 3-4 day a week full-body 60-minute cardio routine that I frequently use in the gym for strength and cardiorespiratory endurance. I rotate lower and upper body exercises first in the workout every other day. I use six different exercises for 10 minutes each while maintaining a constant steady-state of 80-85% for an hour.

1. Stationary bike: resistance level 15; distance 3 miles; time 8:30; RPM 90-100.

2. Arm cranker: resistance level highest; both arms 5 minutes; each arm for 30 second intervals for 5 minutes.

3. Stairmill: speed level 10; execution: knee flexion, good posture, arms free.

4. Battle ropes: I rotate between three movements: single waves, double waves, and hulk smashes.

5. Elliptical: resistance level 14; execution: mini-squat, knee flexion, arms free, no momentum or bouncing upper body; distance 1+ miles; 7mph.

6. 8 lb. dumbbells (300 reps): Front raises 25 → Side raises 25 → Landmine presses 25 → Bicep curls 25 → Dumbbell rows 25 → Tricep kickbacks 25 → REPEAT

APPENDIX B-1

RESISTANCE TUBE TRAINING ROUTINE
COVID-19 LOCKDOWN

I did not stop training during COVID-19 lockdown. This is the 3-4 day a week full-body 60-minute resistance tube routine that I used at home to continuing training. I used three tubes: blue (40 lbs.), red (30 lbs.), and green (20 lbs.). I rotated upper or lower body first in my workout every other day.

<u>Upper body warm-up</u> (red tube): 300 reps in 8 minutes
Front raises 25 → Side raises 25 → Landmine presses 25 → Bicep curls 25 → Rows 25 → Tricep kickbacks 25 → REPEAT

<u>Upper body</u>
Chest (burnsets: 1 & 2)
1. Push-ups on fists (elbows in) 45, 25
2. Chest flys (all tubes) anchored in door, leaning forward, and with staggered stance 30, 20
3. Landmine presses (blue & red) 2 x 15 OR
   Pullovers (all tubes) lying on floor 20, 15

Shoulders (blue) (burnsets: 4 & 5)

4. Front raises (mid to top) 25
5. Front raises (bottom to mid) 25
6. Side raises (bottom to mid) 25
7. Rotator cuff exercise 5 lbs. for 25

Lats (all tubes) (burnsets)

8. Rows 2 x 25
9. Stiff-arm pulldowns 2 x 25

Rhomboids and rear shoulders (burnsets)

10. Reverse flys (blue) elbows bent, pulling in 2 x 20
11. Reverse flys (red) elbows slightly bent, pulling back 2 x 20

Biceps & Triceps (superset)

12. Curls (blue & red) 25, 20, 15
13. Dips on front bed board with feet elevated 45, 40, 35

Lower body warm-up: 3 minutes

Leg extensions (all tubes) 2 x 25 (pause/hold at top)

Lower body

Quads

14. One-leg squats holding onto doorway leaning back 4 x 25 (200 reps in 8 minutes) OR Leg extensions (all tubes) 4 x 25 (30 second rests)

Hams & Abs (burn-supersets: 15 & 16, 15 & 17, 15 & 18)

15. Hamstring curls with exercise ball 3 x 50
16. Reverse crunches with exercise ball 1 x 50
17. Crunches on exercise ball 1 x 50
18. Leg raises exercise ball pass 1 x 20

Calves

19. One-leg standing calf raises on chair 3 x 20

APPENDIX B-2A

CARDIO TUBE TRAINING ROUTINE
COVID-19 LOCKDOWN

This is the 3-4 day a week full-body 60-minute cardio tube routine that I used at home to continue training for strength and cardiorespiratory endurance. I used the blue (40 lbs.) tube exclusively for training upper body for a total of 900 reps. I rotated upper or lower body first in my workout every other day.

Upper body: 8-minutes

    A. Front raises 25 → Side raises 25 → Landmine presses 25 → Curls 25 → Rows 25 → Kickbacks 25 → REPEAT

Lower body: 10 minutes

    B. Wall-sits: 4 minutes

        Box steps: 2 minutes

        Wall-sits: 4 minutes

Upper body: 8 minutes

    A. Front raises 25 → Side raises 25 → Landmine presses 25 → Curls 25 → Rows 25 → Kickbacks 25 → REPEAT

<u>Lower body</u>: 10 minutes

    A. Wall-sits: 4 minutes

        Box steps: 2 minutes

        Wall-sits: 4 minutes

<u>Upper body</u>: 8 minutes

    A. Front raises 25 → Side raises 25 → Landmine presses 25 → Curls 25 → Rows 25 → Kickbacks 25 → REPEAT

<u>Lower body</u>: 10 minutes

    B. Wall-sits: 4 minutes

        Box steps: 2 minutes

        Wall-sits: 4 minutes

APPENDIX B-2B

ALTERNATE CARDIO TRAINING ROUTINE
COVID-19 LOCKDOWN

This is an alternate cardio routine I used for training outdoors on the track at Central Valley High School. I rotated between running up and down steps and running a lap. I sprinted up every other step and briskly walked down each step 10 times for 250 steps as one set. After running up and down the steps, I ran a lap. Distance: 6 miles; Time: 60-minutes.

Step running → Lap running = 1 set/lap
Step running → Lap running = 2 sets/laps
Step running → Lap running = 3 sets/laps
Step running → Lap running = 4 sets/laps
Step running → Lap running = 5 sets/laps
Step running → Lap running = 6 sets/laps
Step running → Lap running = 7 sets/laps
Step running → Lap running = 8 sets/laps
Step running → Lap running = 9 sets/laps
Step running → Lap running = 10 sets/laps

APPENDIX C

HIGH PROTEIN AND LOW CARB
RECIPE DISHES

These are my favorite main dishes that I make for my meals in addition to other foods. For example, shrimp, taco, and chicken salads; zucchini boats and easy enchilada cups (Internet); fried cod breaded fillets; meatloaf hamburger patties; and eggs. I eat few complex carbs, but when I do I get them from flour wheat tortillas.

Cauliflower Pie
Servings: 12

<u>Ingredients</u>
    3 cauliflower heads
    1 lb lean ground beef
    3-4 roma tomatoes (diced)
    1 broccoli stalk (diced)
    A few cut jalapenos from a jar (diced) (for flavor)
    8 oz. Tillamook medium cheddar cheese
    4 heaping Tsp sour cream

1 tsp garlic powder

½ tsp black pepper

<u>Directions</u>

1. Steam cauliflower heads for approximately 60 minutes. Do not overcook to avoid too much moisture. Remove cauliflower and let sit for 5 minutes to cool.

2. Brown ground beef in skillet. Add spices. Steam broccoli but don't overcook. Dice broccoli, tomatoes and jalapenos.

3. Mash cauliflower with potato masher until fine. Add sour cream and stir. Add ground beef, broccoli, tomatoes, and jalapenos. Mix together. Add more sour cream if necessary.

4. Pour half the mix in a 13x9 deep baking dish. Pat it down firmly with the utensil. Grade cheese and layer 5 oz on top. Pour the remaining mix, pat it down, and layer the remaining cheese on top. Bake 350° for 20 minutes.

Cauliflower Pizza

Servings: 12

<u>Ingredients</u>:

3 cauliflower heads

3 eggs

8 Tsp parmesan cheese

1 tsp parsley

8 oz can tomato sauce

8 oz Monterey Jack cheese

8 oz Tillamook medium cheddar cheese

Pepperoni slices

1 can black olives

3-4 tomatoes

<u>Directions</u>:

1. Steam cauliflower heads for approximately 60 minutes. Do not overcook to avoid too much moisture. Remove cauliflower and let sit for 5 minutes to cool. Mash cauliflower with potato masher until fine. Add eggs, parmesan cheese, and parsley. Mix well.

2. Spray cooking sheet with olive oil. Spread half the cauliflower mixture on an aluminum cooking sheet (put the other half in the refrigerator). Cook 350° for 30 minutes. Let sit for a few minutes to cool.

3. Add preferred spices to tomato sauce and lightly spread evenly. Grade cheese and spread 4 oz mixture of Monterey Jack and 4 oz of Tillamook cheddar cheese. Add your preferred toppings. Cook 350° for 15 minutes.

Homemade Chili

Ingredients:

    1 ½ lbs lean ground beef
    4-5 tomatoes (diced)
    3 cans (undrained) kidney beans
    15 oz tomato sauce
    6 oz tomato paste
    2 onions (diced)
    3 jalapenos (diced)

    2 Tsp chili powder
    1 Tsp onion powder
    1 Tsp garlic powder
    1 tsp red cayenne pepper
    2 tsp dried parsley
    1 tsp basil
    ¼ tsp black pepper

Directions:

1. In skillet cook the ground beef. Add beef into crock pot. Sautee onions and jalapenos in the same skillet with olive oil.
2. Mix spices in separate bowl. Add beef, onions, jalapenos and diced tomatoes into crock pot. Add the remaining ingredients and spices. Mix together.
3. Cook low for 4 hours or high for 2 hours (depending on the heating temperature of your crock pot).

Taco Lasagna (tasteofhome.com) – slightly modified

Servings: 12

Ingredients:
  1 lb lean ground beef
  1 green pepper (chopped)
  1 onion (chopped)
  2/3 cup water
  1 envelope taco seasoning
  15 oz can black beans (drained)
  15 oz can diced tomatoes (drained)
  6 flour wheat tortillas (8 inches)
  1 16 oz can refried beans
  8 oz graded Pepper Jack cheese
  8 oz graded Tillamook cheddar cheese

Directions:
  1. In large skillet cook beef until pink before adding the chopped green pepper and onion to the beef. Cook until beef is brown. Add water and stir in taco seasoning. Add black beans, tomatoes and refried beans. Cook on medium heat for 5-10 minutes.
  2. Spread a little bit of the beef mixture on the bottom of greased 13x9 deep baking dish. Place 2 tortillas. Spread with one-third of the mixture. Sprinkle with one-third of the cheese mix. Repeat layers. Top with remaining tortillas, beef mixture and cheese.
  3. Cover and bake at 350° for 25-30 minutes.

Homemade "Mouth-Watering" Burritos

<u>Ingredients</u>:

1 lb lean ground beef
4 oz tomato sauce
1 ½ Tsp catsup
1 Tsp hot sauce
1 Tsp sour cream
1 tsp garlic powder
¼ tsp black pepper
Flour wheat tortillas
Tillamook cheese (graded)
Jar of jalapenos (sliced)
Tomatoes (diced)

<u>Directions</u>:

1. In skillet cook the ground beef. Add tomato sauce, catsup, hot sauce, sour cream, garlic powder, and black pepper. Cook over medium heat for 5 minutes. Simmer.
2. Place the beef mix onto the tortilla and top it with cheese. Microwave 30 seconds to melt cheese.
3. Remove from microwave. Top off the beef and cheese with tomatoes, 3 slices of jalapenos and sour cream.

Reference books for further reading

Aquinas, Thomas. *Commentary on Aristotle's* Nicomachean Ethics (1270). Trans. C. J. Litzinger. Notre Dame: Dumb Ox Books, 1993.

Aristotle, *Nicomachean Ethics* in *The Complete Works of Aristotle,* Vol. 2. Ed. Jonathan Barnes. Princeton: Princeton University Press, 1995.

Briggle, Adam. *A Rich Bioethics.* Notre Dame: University of Notre Dame Press, 2010.

Clark, Nancy. Sports Nutrition Guidebook, 2nd Ed. Champaign: Human Kinetics, 1997.

Csikszentmihalyi, Mihaly. *Flow: The Psychology of Optimal Experience* (1990). New York: Harper Perennial Modern Classics, 2008.

Durant, Will. *The Story of Philosophy* (1926). New York: Pocket Books, 2006.

Emerson, Ralph. W. *The Complete Writings of Ralph Waldo Emerson.* New York: Wm. H. Wise & Co., 1929.

Gardner, Howard. *Intelligence Reframed: Multiple Intelligences for the 21st Century.* New York: Basic Books, 1999.

Gibb, Barry, J. *The Rough Guide to the Brain.* London: Rough Guides, 2012.

Goggins, David. *Can't Hurt Me.* Austin: Lioncrest Publishing, 2020.

Middleton, Christopher (Ed.) *Selected Letters of Friedrich Nietzsche.* Indianapolis: Hackett Publishing, 1996.

Nietzsche, Friedrich. *Untimely Meditations* (1874). Trans. R. J. Hollingdale. Cambridge: Cambridge University Press, 1989.

___. *The Gay Science* (1882). Trans. Walter Kaufmann. New York: Vintage Books, 1974.

___. *Ecce Homo* (1888). Trans. R. J. Hollingdale. London: Penguin Books, 2004.

Parkes, Graham. *Composing the Soul: Reaches of Nietzsche's Psychology.* Chicago: University of Chicago Press, 1994.

Rand, Ayn. *The Virtue of Selfishness.* New York: Signet, 1964.

Stichter, Matt. *The Skillfulness of Virtue: Improving Our Moral and Epistemic Lives* (2018). Cambridge: Cambridge University Press, 2021.

Taylor, C. C. W. (Trans.) *The Atomists: Leucippus and Democritus.* Toronto: University of Toronto Press, 1999.

Tillich, Paul. *The Courage To Be.* London: Yale University Press, 1952.

Endnotes

1. While one may not have body-building per se as a goal, it is still a goal of a body transformation that requires a *similar training process* and mindset as those focused on body-building or body-sculpting.

2. According to the CDC, it was $24 billion around 2000.

3. https://www.cdc.gov/chronicdisease/resources/publications/factsheets/physical-activity.htm

4. https://www.ncbi.nlm.nih.gov/pmc/articles/PMC4779740

5. Patrick, Rhonda. https://www.foundmyfitness.com/episodes/exercise-depression (2019).

6. Gibb, Barry, J. *The Rough Guide to The Brain*, pp. 68-69.

7. Herring, Matthew, P. https://www.pubmed.ncbi.nlm.nih.gov/20177034 (2009).

8. https://www.cdc.gov/nchs/fastats/obesity-overweight.htm (2017-2018).

9. https://www.usatoday.com/story/news/nation-now/2018/06/28/cdc-report-only-23-americans-get-enough-exercise/741433002. The CDC also notes that Americans are still "not getting enough exercise."

10. My thanks to my oldest son for directing me to the foregoing CDC reports.

11. *Nicomachean Ethics* in *The Complete Works of Aristotle, Vol. 2*. Book 10, Chapter 5, Lines 1175a29-1175b23ff. Abbr. NE 10.5.1175a29-1175b23ff.

12. Commentary on Aristotle's *Nicomachean Ethics*. Book 3, Lecture 12, Line 512. Abbr. CANE 3.12.512.

13. NE 10.5.1175b9-11.

14. Ibid., 10.5.1175b15-16, 23.

15. Exercising helps you make better food choices because it changes your mindset about food. See: Joo, J., Williamson, S.A., Vazquez, A.I. *et al.* The influence of 15-week exercise training on dietary patterns among young adults. *Int J Obes* 43, 1681–1690 (2019). https://doi.org/10.1038/s41366-018-0299-3. Here is a summary of the study: https://time.com/5517552/exercise-eat-healthier. Also see an abstract of a similar study in 2020: https://pubmed.ncbi.nlm.nih.gov/31764466. These studies show why exercise is 80% and nutrition is 20%. The former influences the latter.

16. *Rotten*, "Troubled Water." Season 2, Episode 3. Directed by Daniel Ruetenik. Narrated by Latif Nasser. Zero Point Zero Production, Inc., Oct. 2019. Netflix.

17. https://www.worldwildlife.org/threats/water-scarcity.

18. Herring, Randy M. "The Contested Enhancement of Caffeine: A Growing Problem to a 'Natural' Alternative." Advanced Biomedical Ethics. Bill Kabasenche. Washington State University, Pullman, Washington (May 5, 2011) 12pp.

19. Internet sources have conflicting statistics. But it seems that worldwide coffee industry revenues are ten times more than bottled water.

20 Most caffeine supplement powders do not give caffeine content except for a "proprietary blend."

21 Briggle, Adam. *A Rich Bioethics,* p. 70.

22 Recently "health-minded" individuals have created online platforms to accommodate MNRs to people who know nothing or little about them. Be cautious and have a discerning mind before you invest in a website offering nutrition and training services. Look for strategic marketing slogans that arouse your emotions and long and drawn out "success stories" seeking to entice you to jump on the bandwagon. Read reviews before you decide to invest in the service!

23 Although discussed in Chapter 4, and applicable to many areas of living, Aristotle's guide to the mean can throw light on finding a macronutrient ratio between the extremes that is right for you and your performance goal.

24 Nietzsche's subtitle to his autobiography and the last book he wrote: *Ecce Homo* (1888).

25 *Untimely Meditations,* "Schopenhauer as Educator," Section 1. Abbr. UM S1.

26 Letter to his friend and theologian Franz Overbeck in 1882. Quoted in *Selected Letters of Friedrich Nietzsche.* Christopher Middleton (Ed.) p. 197. Abbr. SLFN. See Emerson's essay "History," in *The Complete Writings of Ralph Waldo Emerson,* p. 128. Abbr. RWE.

27 UM S1.

28 Nietzsche's 1883 concept of the Overman is most likely derived from the influence of Emerson's 1841 essay "The Over-Soul." See RWE, p. 206. In an 1881 letter to Franz Overbeck, Nietzsche writes that he had become an Emerson enthusiast and he felt Emerson to be a "brother-soul." Quoted in *Composing the Soul* by Graham Parkes, p. 37.

29 *Genius of the Modern World,* "Nietzsche." Directed by Anna Cox. Narrated by Bettany Hughes. Reference commentary by Bettany Hughes. BBC Four, 2016. Netflix; Quoted in SLFN, p. 199.

30 Ibid. Reference commentary by Dr. Manuel Dries of The Open University.

31 Ibid.

32 UM S1 (my emphasis).

33 NE 2.4.1105b5-11.

34 NE 1.7.1098a18-19.

35 *The Story of Philosophy,* p. 98 n. 50. Durant paraphrases NE 2.4. This quote is often misattributed to Aristotle.

36 This idea derives from Ayn Rand's Introduction in *The Virtue of Selfishness.*

37 Stichter, Matt, *The Skillfulness of Virtue,* p. 13. Abbr. TSV.

38 TSV, pp. 13-14.

39 Ibid., 12.

[40] Ibid.

[41] Ibid.

[42] Self-satisfaction, i.e., feeling good about yourself, is the number one reason why people exercise or engage in an activity.

[43] TSV, p. 94

[44] I had originally entitled this chapter and this skill "repetitive instants." But when I was reading Matt Stichter's *The Skillfulness of Virtue* one evening it was by chance that I came across a similar idea that describes this same activity but more precise and inclusive. I decided to adopt "flow experiences" instead of "repetitive instants" because the latter seemed somewhat choppy and rough rather than smooth and calm. The difference for me is a semantical one. See TSV, p. 96ff. Matt Stichter was my thesis director at Washington State University.

[45] Flow experiences can be applied in any sport, activity, pleasure, career or intellectual pursuit to help make life more enjoyable and meaningful.

[46] Quoted in TSV, p. 96ff.; Csikszentmihalyi, Mihalyi. *Flow*, p. 92.

[47] TSV, pp. 96-97, my emphasis.

[48] Ibid.

[49] Ibid., 54.

[50] Ibid., 73.

[51] Ibid., 90. The word in definition is "autotelic," which is a person who is internally driven and intrinsically motivated with a sense of purpose; auto = self, telic = goal.

[52] Ibid., 72.

[53] Ibid., 58.

[54] You don't have to run to get a runner's high. A runner's high is triggered by any kind of intense cardio *endurance exercise* and training at a steady-state of 80-85% of your maximum heart rate for 45 minutes.

[55] https://appliedpsychologydegree.usc.edu/blog/to-multitask-or-not-to-multitask; https://www.cnn.com/2015/04/09/health/your-brain-multitasking/index.html.

[56] This third habit is directly related to and is the effect of the seventh habit "adaptation" in Chapter 7.

[57] Cycling means exerting a "level of effort" *relative to your* highest intensity. Training 'intensity' is briefly mentioned below and described in Chapter 5.

[58] Resting between 30-90 seconds is a good medium range for building muscular endurance and losing fat (30 s) and gaining muscle (90 s). The relationship between muscle recovery and time ranges from 15.4% after 5 s and 50% after 2 m. See Yates, J. W., Kearney, J. T., Noland, M. P. et al. "Recovery of dynamic muscular endurance." *Europ. J. Appl. Physiol.* 56, 662-667 (1987) https://doi.org/10.1007/BF00424807. This is why a 5 s rest/pause allows you to perform a rep or two more than if you performed the reps "non-stop," which forces the muscles to fatigue quicker in order to stimulate the potential for more muscle faster.

59 *Sports Nutrition Guidebook,* p. 191. Abbr. SNG.

60 Ibid., 197.

61 Ibid., 195.

62 Elaine McGee, RD (2011). "Chocolate Milk vs. Recovery Drinks: Which One Comes Out on Top?" WebMD. https://blogs.webmd.com/from-our-archives/20110817/chocolate-milk-vs-recovery-drinks-which-one-comes-out-on-top.

63 Ibid.; SNG, pp. 195-6, especially Table 11.1.

64 NE 2.2.1103b31.

65 Ibid., 2.2.1104a9.

66 Paul of Tarsus had a kind of athletic mindset. Like a fitness coach, he admonishes his audience to be "temperate in all things;" so they may "run in such a way" as one who competes to obtain *"the prize."* 1 Cor. 9:22-27.

67 Goggins, David. *Can't Hurt Me,* p. 140.

68 Tillich, Paul, *The Courage To Be,* p. 28.

69 *The Gay Science* (1882), Section 382, his emphasis. Abbr. GS.

70 There is no reason why you should take an extreme course of action and decrease your workout intensity because of wearing a face mask. Challenge yourself and think of it as "altitude training" and train harder. Altitude training simply reduces the amount of air flow to the lungs. The benefit of wearing a face mask (and once you stop wearing one) is that your strength, muscle and endurance will be improved. It's the resolve to push through pending obstacles by *adapting to demanding circumstances* for the thrill of *your* victory!

71 Venturing off into the wild for a deeper appreciation of nature can be a good thing but not at the extreme course of action taken by Chris McCandless. Chris' adventures in the Alaskan Wilderness in 1992 in recounted in Jon Krakauer's book *Into The Wild* (1996) and made into a 2007 film.

72 A bicycle ride from Newport Beach at Jamboree Road and San Joaquin Hills Road to Venice Beach, Gold's Gym is 53 miles and takes four and half hours.

73 The well-known quote "Do not go where the path may lead; go instead where there is no path and leave a trail" is often misattributed to Ralph Waldo Emerson.

74 Dr. Howard Gardner expounds his theory of multiple intelligences in *Intelligence Reframed: Multiple Intelligences for the 21ˢᵗ Century.* His theory reinforces "the idea that individuals have many talents that can be of use to society; that a single measure (like high stake test) is inappropriate for determining graduation, access to college etc.; and that important materials can be taught in many ways, thereby activating a range of intelligences" (Email to Randy Herring by Dr. Gardner, May 2003).

75 *The Atomists: Leucippus and Democritus,* D47, p. 21.

[76] RWE, p. 152.

[77] There are several *YouTube* motivational videos featuring Will Smith's perspective on failure noted here verbatim.

[78] Quote by Fred DeVito.

[79] There are several *YouTube* motivational videos featuring Will Smith's perspective on self-love noted here verbatim.

[80] See Chapter 8.

[81] See the Introduction and Chapter 1.

[82] See the Introduction.

[83] Adapted and modified from: https://www.self.com/story/signs-of-successful-workout.

[84] Arnold's successor, 3x Mr. Olympia Frank Zane, used high-volume with light weight and high reps. He trained twice a day and exercised each muscle group two to three times a week. He is classified as an ectomorph and most likely has a predominance of slow-twitch muscle fibers (type I).

[85] Durell, Dave. "Effective Strength Training: Understanding the Intensity-Duration Relationship" (1999) at: https://www.naturalstrength.com/2012/12/effective-strength-training.html (2012). It is interesting to note that the ESPN/Gold's Gym unpublished study in 1993 sets the stage and context of the mid to late 90s Great Debate between Arnold and Dorian regarding high-volume vs high-intensity training in 1997. Dorian Yates was the reigning Mr. Olympia from 1993 to 1997.

[86] The planes of motion image is credited to CC BY-SA 4.0 at https://creativecommons.org/licenses/by-sa/4.0. The image was modified by removing two of the three names of planes (as noted by arrow) in order to emphasize each plane of motion discussed.

[87] Sources to assist in explaining the planes of motion including the exercises involved derive from ACE: https://www.acefitness.org/fitness-certifications/ace-answers/exam-preparation-blog/2863/the-planes-of-motion-explained; and NASM: https://blog.nasm.org/exercise-programming/sagittal-frontal-traverse-planes-explained-with-exercises.

[88] Disclaimer: I am not a kinesiologist. Exercise descriptions are based on my *National Academy of Sports Medicine* (NASM) personal training knowledge.

[89] Exercise drawings are credited to Everkinetic at http://db.everkinetic.com; CC BY-SA 4.0 at https://creativecommons.org/licenses/by-sa/4.0. No changes were made with the drawings. Some drawings that were not available to match my text descriptions are clearly noted "unlike the drawing." I chose to stay with the same drawings because they are faceless and exhibit a mainstreamed athlete performing the exercises in relatively good form.

90   Do not place your joints in a position where you know they cannot physically go because of an injury or limitation. The beautiful thing about "free-floating resistance" is that you can manipulate the movement (unlike a machine – one size fits all) that best feels good and safe for you.

91   Describing some joint alignment and body positions for exercises might overlap with ROM.

92   Parallel bar dips can be used for either the chest, front shoulders and triceps muscles. Triceps are worked when the body is more vertical to the floor and elbows in toward the midline of the body. Front shoulders are worked when the body is leaning forward as much as possible. The chest is worked when the body is in the middle position (like Aristotle's golden mean) between working the front shoulders and triceps.

93   The function of the trapezius muscle is to elevate and depress the shoulder blades. The function of the lat muscles is to draw back and pull in (retract) the shoulder blades.

94   This is the secret to "peaking-out" the biceps and working them fully.

95   45-degrees is understood when observing the arm from midpoint (horizontal) position to the floor to the stopping point at 45-degree full flexion.

96   The lats have many functions depending on the position of the body. I have limited its function in respect to the positions of pulldowns and rows.

97   A very wide grip will prevent a full ROM and contracted position because the arms are further away from the body.

98   To keep the elbows forward and in alignment with the upper body simply pivot the shoulder joint back to move the elbow joint forward. The shoulder cannot be in alignment since the bar is pulled down in front of the neck.

99   The erector spinae muscle consists of three long muscles and tendons that originates from the top of the vertebrae at T12 and inserts all the way down to the bottom of the vertebrae at T1. That is, from the base of the human skull to the base of the pelvis.

100   Every so often rotate these hand grips. For example, one month take a left underhand grip and a right overhand grip. Next month take a right underhand grip and a left overhand grip. This can help avoid muscle imbalances or an injury to a rhomboid muscle by weakening one side if you constantly use the same overhand grip with the same hand for many years.

101   Fabio Comana (2010). "Is it ever okay for your knees to extend beyond your toes while squats or lunges?" Ace Fitness. https://www.acefitness.org/education-and-resources/lifestyle/blog/562/is-it-ever-okay-for-your-knees-to-extend-beyond-your-toes-while-doing-squats-or-lunges.

[102] Some fitness enthusiasts are taught by trainers to complete a barbell squat into a full knee and hip extension with a forward hip thrust. This does two ineffective things: removes the constant tension in the quads and hips and deactivates a neutral spine position increasing risk of injury.

[103] I read this on a website: "Most fitness experts and coaches advise people to not use an isolating Leg Extension Machine due to the unnatural pressure it places on the knees and ankles. Regular use of the machine can lead to permanent knee injuries." Nothing can be further from the truth. Who are these "fitness experts and coaches" that this website references? Leg Extensions *build* muscle and *strengthen* tendons and ligaments around the knee joint to keep it strong. Leg Extensions do not weaken the knees and are not the *cause* of knee injuries. What causes weak knees or knee injuries is the kind of exercise modality a person engages in and how he or she uses a particular exercise. What causes knees injuries are high-impact *exercising* and being overweight. Weight resistance training exercise is low-impact bar none. You are in control of your environment, not the other way around.

[104] Exercise ball hamstring curls using a lat pulldown machine is one of my favorites. See https://www.youtube.com/watch?v=84W26sLt_UI

[105] The standing calf raise machine can be an excellent alternative for exercising the trapezius or trap muscles. Simply lower the shoulder pad height and stand on the floor. Place the pads under your shoulders and elevate the traps by shrugging the shoulders.

[106] Performing spinal flexion movements (ab training) after heavy compound movements like squats and deadlifts is recommended to stretch and relax the lumbar spine and for a strong balanced core.

[107] I have omitted horizontal flexion and rotation movements because, although they are important for keeping the shoulder strong and mobile, I reserved myself to more common movements of the shoulders in weight training.